DEATH of COMPASSION

DEATH of COMPASSION

The endangered doctor-patient relationship

Jeffrey Thurston, M.D.

First published in the United States of America in 1996 by WRS Publishing, a division of WRS Group, Inc., 701 N. New Road, Waco, Texas 76710
Book design by Georgia Brady
Jacket design by Joe James

10 9 8 7 6 5 4 3 2 1

Library of Congress Catalog Card Number

ISBN 1-56796-119-3

To Lynne, Kelly, and Andy,
whose willing sacrifice of what little time
they have with Daddy made this book possible

CONTENTS

FOREWORD

SOMETHING IS HAPPENING to American health care. It's been happening for some time now. Right before our eyes. As national attention is focused on containing spiraling health-care costs, the hidden price of that containment eats away at the heart of our medical delivery system. The price of containment may be the doctor-patient relationship unless the danger of its erosion is recognized and certain misguided attempts at reform are redirected.

In more than fifty years of surgical practice, I have been dismayed at the recent escalating, tragic conflict between medical and financial priorities. As president and chairman of the Department of Surgery at Baylor College of Medicine for many years, and now as its chancellor, I have supervised the training of thousands of physicians. The disparate goals of physicians who were trained to put the patient's welfare first and those of the profit-driven, insurance-owned medical corporations are rapidly disillusioning physicians and patients alike. Increasingly, the sanctity of life is being subordinated to Mammon, and medical decisions are being dictated by those unqualified to do so. The patient's choices are being wrested, and the physician's authority is being expropriated—to the detriment of all.

If, in 1956, we had had the same commercial environment that we have today, we might never have developed the heart-lung machine that launched open-heart surgery, or synthetic aortic grafts, or mechanical assist devices for the failing heart, or any of a myriad of medical miracles that derived from the research of the academic medical centers of excellence. Today our teaching institutions are threatened financially by the changing third-party payment system and the evaporation of research funds. In that environment, where will we find the answers to currently incurable diseases?

Dr. Thurston explores these issues with actual patient histories, firsthand accounts of the frustrations and dangers involved in profit-motivated, corporate medicine.

Often with satirical wit, sometimes with heart-rending depictions of utter anguish, his stories unfold with the same fascination as an intriguing novel.

While recognizing a need for some reform in our health system, Dr. Thurston opens our eyes to the dangers of "reforms" based solely on cost-containment. Managed care may be here, but as it develops, we need to make certain that the interests of the patient remain paramount rather than being relegated to an obscure footnote.

As the self-appointed health-policy "experts" continue to bombard the public with their ill-conceived but superficially seductive "health reforms," it is imperative that the public be alerted to the dire consequences to the nation's health and economy that will ensue. So turn the page and get an insider's view of a physician's world in 1995. Experience a glimpse of his training and of the cases that have shaped him as a person and a physician. But most of all take heed, because something disquieting is happening in the world of medicine. And when you experience its effects, you may not like it.

—MICHAEL E. DEBAKEY, M.D.
Chancellor and Distinguished
Service Professor of Surgery
Director, DeBakey Heart Center
Baylor College of Medicine
Houston, Texas
1995

ACKNOWLEDGMENTS

I OWE A TREMENDOUS DEBT of gratitude to my editor, Chris Tucker, who, from the moment of his involvement with this book, taught me that organization is at least as important as content. He proved an invaluable sounding board and a tremendously insightful commentator. This work would not have come to fruition without his continued faith and support.

My thanks to Thomas Spence, president of WRS Publishing, for his patience and thoroughness, as well as to Jonathan Doddridge and Georgia Brady.

I wish to thank all of those at WRS and especially Dr. Wayman R. Spence for believing that there was something here that needed to be said and, more importantly, needed to be heard.

I would like to thank both Baylor College of Medicine in Houston and the University of California in San Francisco for their outstanding programs which allowed me to enter the field of my choice with a very solid clinical background.

I cannot forget my parents, without whose consistent love, support, and teaching I would not be who I am. I also owe a debt of gratitude to my big brother, Scott. In our childhood he bested me in every contest, physical and mental, as older brothers are prone to do. It was that competition in "brotherly love" which helped me to develop the willpower necessary for achieving my goals.

I also wish to recognize the support of Edwin M. Stone, M. D., Ph.D., who has been my best friend and trusted counselor for almost twenty years.

My partners—Drs. B. Henry Estess, Jr., David Bookout, James Richards III, John D. Bertrand, and Bernadine Bank—deserve my gratitude as well. Their patience, constant support, and reliable coverage have contributed to this work.

It goes without saying, but it needs to be said, that this work would not have been possible without the constant support and guidance of God Almighty in the person of his Son, my personal Lord and Savior.

Acknowledgments

Lastly, I would like to thank all those women out there who answer the question "Who's your doctor?" by giving my name. It is not only for your benefit that I write this book, but because of you that I feel so strongly. For the physician, his patients are his strength, his inspiration, his reason for living. They are, in fact, who he is.

INTRODUCTION

I USED TO BE A DOCTOR. You know, a physician. Someone who had patients that he cared for, looked after. Someone to whom people came for help because they didn't feel good or they were scared or they were confused or injured.

No longer. Now they tell me I'm a "health-care provider." I no longer have patients, because people like you, who used to be patients, have become customers. You know, like, "I'm sorry, lady, you can't return the blouse just because you look lousy in it. Now move along, please, we've got lots of folks in line."

I'm a thirty-nine-year-old obstetrician-gynecologist at a major private institution in Dallas, Texas. I came to this startling sense of enlightenment in late 1993 at one of the new breed of seminars, this one dealing with "managed care" and presented by a short, balding, gray-headed man with a goatee.

Mr. Goatee represented one of the huge, omnipotent companies in the health insurance industry, the name of which you would no doubt recognize. Over the course of an hour and a half, he proceeded to lecture two hundred physicians on the inevitable changes to be wrought by impending health-care reform. These changes, he declared in a condescending tone, were to be imposed upon us from the "outside" and we would finally have to conduct our "business" like every other "organized human activity," with higher regard for "purchaser satisfaction."

Now it is roughly three o'clock in the morning, several weeks after the seminar at which I was baptized into my new identity as health-care provider. That may seem like an unusual time for the creative spirit to move me, but I do most of my writing while on call at the hospital. New babies don't always schedule their arrivals between the hours of nine and five, and that means plenty of waiting. Time to think.

This night, as I wait for Mother Nature once again, I'm thinking about what Mr. Goatee said. It occurred to me then, as I'm sure it did to others, that he hadn't the slightest idea what he was talking about. He may know his own business, but he has no idea what a physician is or does or believes, or what might be involved in becoming one.

And this gentleman was supposed to be an expert on health-care reform. He represents the insurance industry, which is far more influential than the federal government in driving reform.

No doubt Mr. Goatee and his corporate cohorts would have their own definition of managed care and its sibling, managed competition. To me, they are umbrella terms for a widespread health-care delivery system in which decisions about diagnosis and treatment are no longer made solely in the best interest of the patient by those most capable of making those decisions. Instead, the decisions are made by persons whose goal is the profitability of the payor. Patients are just now starting to realize that, while their company's new health plan looked good initially with that $10 co-pay, they have very limited options as to where and from whom they can seek their health care.

Most of the doctors at that seminar know that the practice of medicine differs markedly from the selling of small appliances or used cars. But what about our patients? (I mean customers.) As I thought back on what Mr. Goatee had said, I wondered how many Americans he spoke for with his demands that we physicians must practice medicine by focusing on "purchaser [i. e., insurer] satisfaction" and conduct our "business" like every other "organized human activity."

I don't know the answer to that question. The opinion polls tell us many things, but they don't tell us that. But I do know this: If Mr. Goatee's views are held by any significant portion of the American public, then a vast gulf has opened up between physcians and patients. Something has gone terribly wrong.

It is said that America has the best health-care system in the world. I believe it is true, not just because of the money we put into our system, or the high-tech machines that help us perform everyday miracles, but because of something even more important: the doctor-patient relationship, which depends on two related freedoms.

In that relationship, as we have long recognized it, the patient is free to choose his or her doctor and facility. This freedom to choose forms the foundation of our market economy and our very nation. True freedom to choose breeds self-correction in the health-care marketplace just as in other marketplaces.

Second, the doctor, by virtue of what he has learned both academically and in the trenches (and, I hope, by virtue of his resulting wisdom), earns not just the intellectual authority, but the *moral* authority to care for patients. Where a patient's well-being is concerned, the combination of the patient's input and the doctor's expertise should make his decision inviolate.

So-called managed care, as it is already evolving even without government intervention, is severely altering the doctor-patient relationship, transforming what can be a very special personal interaction into a business transaction. It is usurping the doctor's decision-making power, forcing diagnostic and treatment decisions to be made by a third party whose central concern is cost.

How could we as a country have come to this point? Is it the medical profession's fault? Perhaps in our occasional haste, our frequent arrogance, our all-too-visible wealth, we doctors have alienated our patients to the point that they will sacrifice the physician-patient relationship.

Perhaps we drifted apart because the doctor-patient relationship is necessarily one-sided. We physicians are privy to all manner of intimacies gleaned from a patient's health history, but the patient rarely hears anything about the physician's private trials and tribulations. We learn something about the person you are and what has brought you to this moment, but you learn little about who we are and what shaped us.

Some aspects of the health-care system are in dire need of reform—but some of the proposed "cures" would destroy the greatest health-care system the world has ever seen. As we seek to alter the health-care system in America, we should heed the Hippocratic aphorism *Primum non nocere*—First, do no harm.

I want to talk about how to change the system later,

but that is just one of my reasons for writing this book. I also want to talk about something that entirely escaped the seminar speaker, Mr. Goatee, and seems to be missing from the debate over reform.

I want to communicate something of what it means to be a physician. That, more than any direct argument I can make against managed care, will *show* you, not just tell you, why it is a grave error to allow the usurpation of the physician's moral and clinical authority by any outside agency.

Now it would be impractical for a doctor to take up a patient's valuable time during an office visit to tell his own life story or complain about the new hurdles that complicate a doctor's work today. But estrangement is usually born of misinformation, as are prejudice and envy and violence. If people are misinformed about the physician in general and about the ways in which managed care is already affecting the quality of their care, then we as doctors should strive to make them better informed.

In this book you will get a better understanding of what is involved in becoming a doctor. I also want to share with you the paradox of the doctor-patient relationship. While the patient comes to the doctor in need of his scientific expertise and guidance, it is you, the *patient*, who teaches the vital courses in humanity that supplement the doctor's science. The physician's training, coupled with these life lessons, puts him in the best position to help you make decisions about your health care.

You will also get a glimpse of the frustrations and, ultimately, the dangers entailed in grossly restricting— and finally removing—the doctor's decision-making authority and limiting the patient's freedom to choose a doctor. If we destroy the physician-patient relationship, the very heart of American medicine, our society will be traveling a perilous road indeed.

Finally, you'll be able to consider some possible solutions to the system's very real problems. Unlike the remedies of managed competition, these proposed solutions neither destroy the physician's effectiveness and desire, nor restrict the patient's ability to choose her own caregiver.

All of the following stories are true. You will find some of these stories sad, some funny, some poignant, and some gruesome, but each played its part in my development as a physician.

I hope this book helps you understand physicians better and to know that the best doctors become what they are by listening to patients. I've tried to listen. Here is what I've learned.

WELCOME TO THE SINCERE HEALTH-CARE NETWORK. IF YOU ARE A DOCTOR OR A HOSPITAL CALLING, PLEASE...

PRESS 1 AND THE # SIGN NOW

IF YOU ARE CALLING TO INQUIRE ABOUT
YOUR PREMIUMS OR ACCOUNT STATUS...

PRESS 2 AND THE # SIGN NOW

IF YOU ARE CALLING TO INQUIRE ABOUT
PRECERTIFICATION FOR AN IN-PATIENT
PROCEDURE OR TO OBTAIN AN
OUT-PATIENT REFERRAL NUMBER...

PRESS 3 AND THE # SIGN NOW

IF YOU ARE CALLING TO INQUIRE ABOUT A CLAIM, REPORT AN ERROR, OR ARE RETURNING A CALL FROM US...

PRESS 4 AND THE # SIGN NOW

IF YOU HAVE SELECTED ANY OF THE
NUMBERS 1 THROUGH 4 IN THE
PREVIOUS MENU...

PLEASE HOLD

IF YOU ARE FRUSTRATED, CONFUSED, ANGRY, OR SIMPLY WANT TO SEE *YOUR OWN* DOCTOR,

TURN THE PAGE NOW...

SEEING MUCH, SUFFERING MUCH,
AND STUDYING MUCH,
THESE ARE THE THREE PILLARS OF LEARNING.

—BENJAMIN DISRAELI

PART ONE

SEEDS OF COMPASSION

WHILE IN COLLEGE, I had almost no idea of what might be involved in medical school above and beyond diligent study. My life from birth to about twenty-one did very little to prepare me for the bizarre experiences I would have while training to be a physician.

Looking back on those years, I now realize that some of those experiences shaped the course of future events for me—in fact, they shaped the person that I am. All physicians have similar anecdotes, the "war stories" one used to hear in physicians' lounges before managed care and medical-legal issues came to dominate the conversation.

The lessons begin very early on. They plant the seeds of compassion. They make it possible to "suffer with" the patient, in the literal sense of the word "compassionate." These lessons often contribute more to the future doctor's character than to his fund of knowledge. But that character is the foundation of the physician-patient relationship. In turn, that relationship, combined with scientific knowledge, puts the physician in the best position to make the decisions that most benefit those patients whose sacred trust he has sworn to uphold.

1

SEVENTEEN

UNTIL RECENTLY, ALL MEDICAL SCHOOL candidates had to be in the top 1 to 5 percent of their undergraduate classes. While remaining in this elite group may seem a substantial challenge in and of itself, most of us left high school pretty sure of our abilities. All of us were, by definition, at the top of our high school classes and saw no reason why that should change at the college level.

What many of us did not realize is that a lot of those students we left in the academic dust had never intended to go on to college, so beating them to the finish line was a pretty hollow victory. Furthermore, many private universities had a way of concentrating the best and the brightest within their hedges. In short, many of us who would eventually enter medical school were about to have our initial experience with real competition, and first prize was a lesson in humility.

A perfectly good number really, seventeen. Could be good as the chapter number, the number of years I've been in medicine, the age at which the opposite sex was an all-consuming interest, the number of billions that the federal government borrows in a month, the number of games the Dallas Cowboys won in the '92–'93 season, the age of my Siamese cat, or any of a myriad of other things.

It is not, however, a particularly good number to have written boldly in red across the top of one's first chemistry test at Rice University.

Now the public perception of physicians may have changed in many ways over the last thirty or forty years, but in some ways it remains unaltered. In general, most would agree that medical doctors are not dummies. Admittedly, some may have the bedside manner of John Madden, but they're not supposed to be stupid. Even your average high-school student knows that you're not supposed to see numbers like seventeen written on anything you ever do, especially if you wish to one day have the initials M.D. after your name.

In short, racking up a seventeen was not a step in the proverbial right direction. But before you conclude that if in fact I was making seventeens on my freshman chemistry tests, perhaps I should not focus a KTP laser in your pelvic cavity, a little background information is warranted.

Rice University's incoming freshman class of 1974 was over 70 percent National Merit Scholars and over 60 percent valedictorians. Although only salutatorian in my highly regarded private high school, I could at least lay claim to National Merit Scholarship. I had placed out of biology, calculus, and English and was taking chemistry only because I knew that inorganic, then organic, then biochemistry would be required by most medical schools. (I wasn't convinced at this point that I wanted to be a physician, but I wanted to leave all the doors open.) In short, I thought, as did most of the others, that I was pretty hot stuff academically.

It took exactly nine class days for Rice to make clear that "hot stuff" was a relative term. Lo and behold, there were people from all over this country with considerably more cerebral firepower than *moi*.

Seventeen. *Seventeen?* Of course at first I assumed this was the percentage I had gotten incorrect. Well, that's not so bad... Wrong, *mon ami!* Next I assumed that the test would be graded on a curve. Wrong yet again, *mon cheri!* In the vernacular, I had flunked it—"screwed the pooch," I believe is the immortal term used by astronaut Gus Grissom after his Gemini capsule sank.

There was some consolation in my discovery that 17 percent was the third-highest grade in the class. It remained, however, my first academic failure. Not unlike many pre-med students in fact, for the first time in my life I had received a grade other than an A. (Uh, except for the C I received in—and this is the God's honest truth—handwriting in the third grade.)

This may seem silly to you non-anal-retentive, non-compulsive types, but we pre-meds saw it as a big deal at

4

the time. You just don't get seventeens. It just flat out does not happen. Denial, remorse, fear, anger, etc., all apply here. Elizabeth Kubler-Ross, author of *On Death and Dying,* would have put this somewhere between losing your spouse and children beneath an overturned cement truck and the annihilation of life as we know it in a nuclear holocaust. Your whole life flashes before your eyes. Forget being a doctor. Forget being an engineer. No more possibility of a lucrative career as a small animal vet. Hell, with a seventeen on your record, would a law school even take you?

Well, time heals all wounds, and as I flunked tests in multiple other disciplines I began to feel much better. This was clearly part of the plan. If it was intended to catch the students' attention and get their noses to the grindstone, we were all down to the cartilage in a matter of weeks.

But like so many other experiences that seem like disasters at the time, this event too shaped the future physician. A little humility goes a long way with colleagues and patients alike. Rice University and that chemistry professor had made a contribution to the humility fund right from the git-go.

Humility, of course, has long been viewed as an essential virtue of the well-rounded character. Ben Franklin added it to his list of virtues to be actively attained and in fact did so well that, in his *Autobiography,* he reports being "quite proud of my humility." He could have been a doc!

YONNIE

OTHER THAN TELEVISION and their own limited encounters with emergency rooms for broken arms and the like, most college students have no exposure to medicine at all. Often their introduction to the real world of medicine involves a job which takes them into limited contact with doctors, nurses, technicians, and patients.

Some students work as orderlies or clerks. I got an unusual job with an extraordinary mentor, and I learned that a slipshod approach to my job might put the technician and physician out of work and kill the patient. That taught me the meaning of the word "responsibility."

Yonnie. In a roundabout way, Yonnie was responsible for the tremendous blow to my forehead which I received at about 4:30 on that particular Monday morning.

The more direct cause lay in my position at the time. I was lying beneath the steel desk with my head no more than six feet from the cow theoretically under surveillance. Sleep had been my companion for only about an hour since my last readings. Suddenly something struck the sole of my left foot, awakening me and instantaneously propelling me into a sitting position.

Unfortunately, the desk did not quite allow adequate clearance for the sitting position and thus the fierce blow to my head only microseconds after my foot had been similarly insulted. Needless to say, I uttered several expletives, college students being particularly adept at this form of expression. I slid myself out from under the desk and looked straight up at my assailant. Even more unfortunately, the guilty party was my employer, an extremely well known six-foot, four-inch cardiothoracic surgeon.

"Who in the heck's watching my cows?" he snapped. I didn't think this was the proper time to remind Dr.

Denton Cooley that they weren't technically *his* cows. After all, it was 4:30 a.m. But if he wanted to make rounds on the cows before the people, that was certainly his prerogative.

If you're at all confused, add to the scenario that this is taking place on the third floor of the Texas Heart Institute in Houston, Texas, in November 1977. I was a pre-med student at the prestigious Rice University across the street, trying to earn a few extra bucks in the Total Artificial Heart (TAH) program. This TAH program, among others like it, was continuing the work of many investigators which would eventually lead to the placement of a permanent artificial heart in Dr. Barney Clark at the University of Utah in 1982. That procedure—and in fact all open-heart procedures—evolved from the pioneering work of Dr. Michael DeBakey. Dr. DeBakey had, in 1932, invented the central component to the heart-lung bypass machine. His later work at Baylor College of Medicine, in conjunction with the Rice Biomedical Engineering Department, led to a temporary mechanical-assist device, or partial artificial heart, implanted as early as 1963 and subsequently refined in the late sixties.

My job was to take the Swan Ganz catheter recordings, administer antibiotics, feed, water, and otherwise nurture two cows whose natural hearts had been replaced with plastic ones that operated pneumatically. (Prior to Barney Clark there were a large number of less famous cows.)

By day I was a mild-mannered biology major at Rice, but by night I was the phantom technician upon which the success or failure of the TAH program firmly rested. Several centers around the world were involved in such research, but the one with which we competed most directly was a very successful group out in Utah.

The Utah folks had calves (little cows, for non-Texans) living for hundreds of days and actually outgrowing their hearts! Our moos had a nasty tendency to die of sepsis or to be sacrificed, as I understood it at the time, in the interests of drug studies for companies who in large part funded the research. We all kinda thought the guys in Utah had an unfair advantage. They were going strictly

7

for longevity records, while our cows had many more holes in their chests for hoses and IVs, and therefore many more opportunities for infection while we studied all kinds of drug effects. Nonetheless, longevity counted, and college students who slept on the job did little to advance the cause.

As it happened, when Denton Cooley caught me snoozing, he was most forgiving and allowed me to rise to my feet and fill him in on the night's events. During my stint that night, I learned not only cardiopulmonary physiology, as usual, but one of my first little lessons about self-discipline. Errors in drug administration or readings could lead to faulty data, or worse, the premature loss of a cow. That could translate into millions of dollars of lost grant money, which could in turn mean people lost their jobs, which down the road could mean sick people lost their lives. All of a sudden I was thankful the good doctor hadn't taken my sleepy head off.

Oh, yes, Yonnie. Yonnie is short for "Yonder" as in "Hither and Yonder." These were the Harlequin Great Danes belonging to Dr. Norman, who was actually in direct charge of the TAH lab. Yonnie spent her nights in the third-floor lab as security and sometime companion. She liked the couch. So did I, but Yonnie weighed 160 pounds, and when she stood on her hind legs, she put her forepaws on my shoulders and looked down at me. She got the couch. I slept on the floor, under the desk.

A BIG PROBLEM

MY FIRST EXPERIENCES with human patients took place only a few hundred yards from the cows in the Texas Heart Institute. Big county emergency rooms are not only the salvation of many of our nation's trauma victims, they're the proving grounds for our physicians-in-training. As such, the medical student comes in contact with family tragedies for the first time, but also with truths that are often stranger than fiction. The following really occurred, and taught me that there is often no dignity in death unless we make it so.

The first two years of medical school are largely didactic and are spent either in a lecture hall or a laboratory of some sort. However, if you wanted an early taste of this doctor stuff, you could work for nothing in the emergency room at night and thus fill the gobs of free time you had available when you eliminated sleep from your agenda. My roommate Ed and I volunteered.

County ERs are the crossroads for every bizarre type of human that you could envisage with a very fertile imagination. Add alcohol, drugs, impatience, sometimes filth, and often animosity, and you have the recipe for some very unusual occurrences. My second night ever in the Ben Taub ER, affiliated with Baylor College of Medicine in Houston, was the setting for this little tragicomedy.

Medical students at my level were essentially worthless to everyone—doctors, nurses, orderlies, and medical technicians. Why? Because we didn't know our ass from a hole in the ground, that's why. We possessed absolutely no knowledge that might be remotely useful in a big-city ER.

So we were asked to go talk to patients who had been waiting for at least ten hours. This could be easily determined by looking for those who had not suffered a gunshot wound to the head or chest and those without protruding knife handles. Some of these moderately sick people were mildly perturbed by the number of shift changes they had witnessed while waiting to be seen.

This particular night I was instructed by one of the residents to take the history of the man in Room 4 with chest pain. I quickly ran by this small room on my way to X-ray on a previously assigned task, intending to peek around the curtain across the doorway and inform the hapless gentleman that someone would be with him in a moment. At a glance I saw no one in the room, just a pair of shoes on the bed.

I delivered the films to X-ray and returned in three to four minutes. To my astonishment, the shoes on the bed turned out on closer inspection still to contain their owner. The patient had fallen over backwards, off the gurney, and lay in an inverted jackknife position (for you swimmers) or just flat crumpled upside down on the floor between the gurney and the wall.

I called down the hall for help and then tried to reach the stricken man. The gurney had been forced away from the wall by the patient's back flip, and was now firmly wedged between an inset column and the door frame. Undaunted, I climbed onto the gurney to peer down at the victim. That's when I clearly understood we had a very serious problem on our hands. This man must have weighed four hundred pounds. (In point of fact, 468 pounds according to the triage nurse's record of his "weight by history.") While he was poorly illuminated in his present locale, he nevertheless looked too damned blue.

Because I was the first to discover this unfortunate situation, others were willing to accord me some proprietary interest in the case and thus elected me to crawl under the gurney and hold an oxygen mask to the man's face. I could find no pulse, but then again I knew very little about where to look. Two residents then tried to force the gurney to an angle where it could be extricated but failed. They then tried to lift it straight up so that the man might flop, as it were, into a lying position and then be dragged out from under the gurney. This likewise failed and in fact worsened the situation in that the man's legs became entangled in the far-side lowered arm rail.

Needless to say, this massively obese gentleman was not doing well. CPR was not physically possible because of his entrapment and would in all likelihood have been ineffectual even had he been lying on the trauma table. About this time the room was also filling with an unbearable odor. Apparently everyone but I knew that this came from the patient and did not suggest a favorable prognosis. In fact, the man was quite dead, but I just couldn't believe it. True, at this point he looked dead enough. But in death there is usually some sense of dignity, is there not?

Perhaps you think me callous to include this anecdote. But all physicians have found themselves in similar black-humor situations during their training, and such situations do play a role in shaping their demeanor.

The incident had another meaning for me. This was the first person I had ever witnessed dying. I had never sat at my great-grandmother's bedside as her life ebbed away, or seen an automobile accident, or found myself at the scene of a drowning or any of a thousand more common scenarios in which people pass away. No, I had to see my first death as an acute myocardial infarction in an inverted 468-pound man wedged in a position where we couldn't help him. He wasn't trapped in the cab of his overturned pickup waiting on the jaws of life to cut him free, he was stuffed between a gurney and a wall in the emergency room, positioned such that absolutely nobody could help him. They had to cut away the door frame with a fire ax to get him out.

I remember clearly going out with the resident to see this man's family. Thank God he had no children, but his parents, brother, and wife were all in the waiting room. They looked just like him. He was here, they told us, for an ingrown toenail. No, he'd never had chest pain to their knowledge. The resident informed them of the forty-six-year-old man's death. Compassion in this case included not elaborating on the exact circumstances of his demise.

11

JANICE

THE DISSECTION OF A CADAVER is a strange and unique experience that leaves a medical student with indelible images and a perspective denied the rest of humanity. It is perhaps only in retrospect that we recognize what we have really learned. True, we learn the details of what a marvelous machine is the human body. But we also learn—through its stark absence—that the soul is who we are. When we treat our living patients, it is perhaps their difference from the cadaver, not their similarity, that guides our decision-making.

As I have suggested already, most of the first two years of medical school involves taking notes and asking questions in a lecture hall. There is, however, some laboratory work. Laboratory work, huh? You visualize glass beakers, Bunsen burners, etched and stained countertops and sinks, bad odors, and just a hint of the gorgeous day outside peeking in through the filthy windows. Right? Well, you get partial credit for the bad odors.

Try thirty naked, dripping, slippery dead people reeking of formalin, all laid out on metal tables. Now imagine hacking away at one of those cadavers for six months.

Mind you, before walking into this lab for the first time, all of us were fairly close to being normal people. By that I mean the only dead people we had seen were impeccably dressed in open caskets, and they were usually people we had held dear. Of course some of us, me included, had never even seen the well-dressed, well-preserved, deceased loved one. Now we were about to learn that medical school was more than note-taking in an auditorium.

None of us had a clue what to expect. I clearly remember walking in and seeing the gleaming metal tables and wondering when and where the actual cadavers came into play. There was the expected skeleton hanging

12

in the corner by the blackboard. There was Carl Harvey, Ph.D., whom we had already come to love as perhaps the outstanding teacher of the basic science curriculum, standing by the blackboard and waving our four-person groups into position at the assigned, numbered stations. The combination of the odor in its eye-watering intensity with the overhead fluorescents (the sole source of illumination) gave the fourth-floor lab the appearance of a large basement somewhere in Transylvania.

Logic, of course, would dictate that the sun be allowed in such a grim place, and maybe even a modicum of fresh air from time to time. Instead, the windows were blacked out with tar paper. No one ever really explained why. Presumably this was done for privacy. Perhaps it was so that any forty-foot-tall relatives of the deceased wouldn't stand a chance of being inadvertently offended? We were to learn, of course, that since morgues are invariably located in the cellar, the interior decorating of this fourth-floor lab would make us feel right at home later in our careers.

My lab partners were Ed, my roommate; Jane, a remarkably attractive blonde (remarkable particularly since she was a fellow Rice alum, and at Rice the admissions process apparently was stacked against pretty girls); and Mark, a handsome Italian-type. On that first day we donned our black aprons and awaited further instructions.

Dr. Harvey informed us that we would be dissecting our cadaver in the order in which neophytes like us could best assimilate information, i.e., easy stuff first. Well, "easy" on a very fat, old, dead lady like ours was definitely extremities first, and upper prior to lower. He also informed us that these bodies were donated to the medical school, either by their owners or their families. It was only common decency that their names not be revealed, but their causes of death could be ascertained by perusing the computer printout by the lab door.

Then it was time to raise our cadavers from the depths. The table tops slid open, and several turns of the crank brought our specimens slowly to the surface. (I knew I'd seen this movie before!) The excess formaldehyde slushed

13

loudly back to the bottom of the metallic table. Some of the less hardy had their eyes closed at this point, anticipating that their donated cadaver would probably have a less pleasing appearance than Aunt Sarah had at the Eternal Rest Funeral Parlor. They needn't have worried, because the donees rose to the surface zipped up in thirty identical black body bags. Why? You might ask. Obviously to keep the smaller parts which were later to be dissected from floating aimlessly and inaccessibly beneath the largely perforated metal sheet which actually rose to support the bodies. Why black? It matched the windows, the aprons, and initially the mood.)

I don't recall which of us had the honor of making the first incisions, but I do recall thinking during the process that perhaps I had made a very serious error in career choice. Somehow I knew that at 10 a.m. on a Monday, there were very few T.I. engineers or G.E. marketing people immersed in similar tasks.

Despite the ghastly appearance of our specimen, with her yellowish gray, slippery skin the texture of shoe leather, her few wisps of gray hair, the incredible weight of her obese, rigid extremities, and that overpowering odor, we decided she would have to have a name. "Our cadaver" was not descriptive enough, and in fact not worthy of this specimen which was not so long ago the repository of a soul. While others named their cadavers in ways that might easily distinguish them from their twenty-nine colleagues (I will not here enumerate the anatomically-related designations at which this group of fertile young minds was able to arrive), we had the misfortune to discover our cadaver's overlooked toe tag. The computer printout had already enlightened us to the age and cause of death (sixty-seven and myocardial infarction, or heart attack—big surprise, I might add) but the tag also revealed her name: Janice Cheops.

Now it was extremely difficult while looking at her in this condition to believe that even distant relatives of hers could have descended from the ancient Egyptian emperors suggested by her surname. Accordingly, the four of us simply adopted the name "Janice" for our cadaver.

Over the course of the next six months, Janice taught

14

us much about the human condition as well as the human body. Obesity became much more of a negative reinforcer for our own health habits, as her liquefying fat made dissection of her corpse infinitely more difficult and disgusting than that of the emaciated old cadaver at the next table over, for example. The carbonization of her lungs by cigarette tar, the cholesterol plaquing of her major arteries, the cirrhotic changes of her liver all served as potent memorials to the dangers of overeating, overdrinking, and underexercising.

After half a year, Janice had become as integral a part of our daily lives as running before work or the minimum three daily showers required to survive the summers in Houston. She was even losing weight gradually, although not by the usual route employed by the living. After removal of the skin came the fat, blood vessels, muscle and tendon, and finally the bones themselves.

The crowning achievement, if you'll excuse the expression, was the opening of the skull, removal of the brain, and study of the attachments of the cranial nerves and associated vasculature—a process difficult enough to make one wonder how someone could have just misplaced President Kennedy's brain. We opened the cranium with a bone saw and lifted off the top of the skull, which then looked just like a Jewish yarmulke.

It was at this juncture that many of us sneaked into the lab on the Saturday before the final exams and obtained a memento of the good times we'd all had together. We used a 35mm Minolta set on timer to create a portrait of Janice in the sitting position, surrounded by her weight-loss management team. Mark, Ed, Jane, and I put on our best smiles while being literally supportive of our teacher.

Now, doing this was strictly against medical school policy. It would be nothing short of disastrous should such a photo ever be seen by the cadaver's loved ones. Not only would it be embarrassing and even cruel, but— who knows?—the family might have donated their relative's money in addition to their relative! We felt sufficiently secure, however, in the knowledge that Janice was, quite frankly, unrecognizable, despite our best efforts to patch her up for the shot. (The editor has recommended that I not include the photograph here and I have deferred to his judgment.)

The reader may think this callous, even bizarre. I think of it now as a way of coping with an experience that I dare say is shared by less than 0.01 percent of the population. Each day, we had to slice into what, for all intents and purposes, was another human being, a creature who had known reason and laughter and tears, and yet our training required us to treat her as no more than a bag of veins, tendons, and muscle—inert meat. We needed humor to lighten the burden. The humor was a shield against the strangeness of it all.

The true desecration was not our humor, but the repeated damage that these corpses' former owners had inflicted on themselves. Our Janice was, in all senses, an empty shell. Her body may once have been a temple, but when the soul departed, it became only a testimony to its defilement, however unintentional, in life.

The images that we physicians take away with us from those anatomy laboratories remain vivid for the rest of our lives. If we fail to see the damage we inflict on our own bodies through lack of sleep, lousy diets, inordinate stress, alcohol, drugs, and cigarettes, perhaps some of us will at least be able to see what those choices are doing to you, by remembering our "Janices."

AEQUANIMITAS

ALL PROFESSIONS HAVE THEIR OWN unique pressures. With few exceptions, however, allowing that pressure to adversely affect performance leads to consequences only for the individual. Physicians, not unlike airline pilots, can kill people when the pressure gets to them.

Some have criticized formal medical-education programs in which medical students and residents work as many as 120 hours per week. They may criticize the public humiliation many students and residents are exposed to in the course of case presentations to more senior physicians. But these are the things that teach the value of evenness under pressure. When you're under the knife, wouldn't you rather know that your physician has been tested by the most adverse physical and emotional circumstances and survived intact?

Aequanimitas is the title of a collection of addresses presented at various places and in various times by the great Sir William Osler, Bt., M.D., F.R.S., professor of medicine, Oxford, and honorary professor of medicine, Johns Hopkins University. Osler delivered the eponymous address of the collection as a valedictory to the University of Pennsylvania Medical School on May 1, 1889.

Aequanimitas, and its English cognate, "equanimity," denote evenness of mind, especially under stress. It is, as Osler points out, regrettable but necessary that a physician, in order to be possessed of equanimity, must distance himself from the emotions that surround the horrors with which he has chosen to deal for the rest of his life, or go mad.

In the first place, in the physician or surgeon no quality takes rank with imperturbability... . Imperturbability means coolness and presence of mind under all circumstances, calmness amid storm, clearness of judgment in moments of grave peril. It is the quality which is most appreciated by the laity though often misunderstood by them... and the physician who has the misfortune to be without it, who betrays indecision and worry, and who shows that he is flustered and flurried in ordinary emergencies, loses rapidly the confidence of his patients.

Professor Osler goes on to say:

From its very nature this precious quality is liable to be misinterpreted, and the general accusation of hardness, so often brought against the profession, has here its foundation. Now a certain measure of insensitivity is not only an advantage, but a positive necessity in the exercise of a calm judgment, and in carrying out delicate operations... Cultivate then, gentlemen, such a judicious measure of obtuseness as will enable you to meet the exigencies of practice with firmness and courage, without, at the same time, hardening "the human heart by which we live."
... the mental equivalent to this bodily endowment [imperturbability] is the watchword, aequanimitas.

If a physician in fact achieves this evenness under pressure, this imperturbability, he may then have some hope of succeeding in his field. Without it, first his patients' confidence fails, and next, of course, his confidence in his own capabilities crumbles as well. All of this probably seems self-evident. But what you might not appreciate is the extreme situations in which this quality of aequanimitas becomes absolutely essential.

I use as an illustration something that happened to a surgical resident and friend of my brother while I was in my second year of basic science. While not, thank God, a firsthand participant, I include this as one of the experiences which colored my medical education.

The resident was working in the county emergency room in the X-ray annex to one of the trauma rooms. The patient lying on the X-ray table was bleeding profusely from an obvious gunshot wound to the upper left thigh. The thigh itself was swollen and discolored. The resident was in the midst of passing a large bore catheter into the groin to be used for injecting radio-opaque dye, a so-called "angiogram." The purpose of this test was to ascertain if in fact the femoral artery had been severed by the bullet, which had passed completely through the leg.

The patient was a big man, dressed in black sweatpants, now opened up the leg with scissors, and a bloody, filthy, formerly white T-shirt. He was semiconscious, rolling his head back and forth and moaning. Other than the female technician across the table from the resident, the only people in the room were two plainclothes police officers positioned near the top of the bed. While the resident was aware that the man was in custody, he was not aware of the crime he allegedly had committed.

Just after the catheter was successfully threaded, while the resident and the technician were watching the fluoroscope monitor at the foot of the bed, one of the plainclothesmen asked whether his prisoner "would make it." Before the surgeon could respond, the small, tiled room reverberated with a tremendous explosion. The technician and the surgical resident jumped up, covering their ears, and turned to see the two plainclothesmen wrestling a uniformed officer to the floor. The patient was no longer moaning. In fact the better part of his skull and its contents were splattered across the leaded-glass wall separating X-ray from trauma. According to my brother, the resident kept his cool, never missing a beat, and answered the officer's question, "Evidently not."

It turned out that the patient had murdered the uniformed officer's partner of eight years. While the resident was obviously shaken by the incident, he did not collapse to the floor in a whimpering heap or run from the room screaming. This truly was imperturbability on a Herculean scale! Not surprisingly, the resident later became a trauma surgeon.

You may ask how anyone could be so unfeeling as to respond to this situation in this way? I ask you how an effective physician could respond in any other way?

There will be many other incidents detailed in the following pages which illustrate this elusive *aequanimitas*.

Many are less gruesome and more poignant, but all involve a doctor's developed ability to separate his natural human responses from the situation and control his temperament and actions.

SURVIVAL
OF THE FITTEST

MENTAL AND EMOTIONAL STRESS are facts of life in the training of the physician from medical school on, and some of that stress is deliberately inflicted in a ritual some may see as cruel. But the doctor-in-training must learn to function on the spot, right that second, sometimes with a life hanging in the balance. Though this trial by fire can be painful and humiliating, the ritual teaches the future doctor to think and act swiftly and precisely.

Samuel Johnson once observed that "when a man knows he is to be hanged in a fortnight, it concentrates his mind wonderfully." So does pimping.

Now don't get the wrong idea. Don't picture girls in leather minis and heavy mascara walking the streets while a diamond-studded business manager lurks in the shadows. As far as any physician I know can remember, the derivation of the term "pimping" is unrelated to the oldest profession.

In the world of medical training, "pimping" refers to the painful ritual wherein one person (usually the ordinate) asks another person (usually the subordinate) a question or series of questions to which there are no specific right answers, thus forcing the subordinate to publicly humiliate himself and either collapse on the floor in a sobbing heap or quietly but noticeably wet his pants.

The medical student is introduced to pimping during study sessions with a classmate. Those of us who were successful at this game recognized early on its essential role in the entire "portal" process. At every level of a doctor's education, from basic sciences to clinical rotations to internship and residency, he must successfully negotiate these rites of passage, and the guardian of the gate is usually called a "pimper."

The highest ranking students quickly figured out how to survive the ongoing pimping ritual that is medical school: Don't think, memorize. If you could memorize the Manhattan phone book over a weekend (and many of us could), you had it made in the shade—thanks in part to cramming sessions propelled by what we called the V-2 Rocket, Vivarin. Why waste time preparing and actually drinking thirty or forty cups of coffee if you can get the equivalent boost more quickly and easily in capsule form? No illegal amphetamines for us, no sir. We just wired ourselves on the V-2 Rocket and we were off, stretching our synapses to the breaking point with vast loads of factoids.

What? Trouble remembering that histamine breaks down into methyl histamine, methylimidazole acetic acid, imidazole acetic acid riboside, imidazole acetic acid and acetylhistamine? Pop another V-2 and read it again while you use your yellow highlighter. (Eventually, every line of every medical school text is highlighted.) Once the task of reading, rereading, and highlighting was completed, the study mates would combine forces and come up with mnemonics that would help them visualize this mass of detail. For example, this little number for the muscles of the medial thigh:

Say	Sartorious
Grace	Gracilis
Before	Semi-membranosus
Tea	Semi-tendinosus

Of course, Vivarin-driven minds sometimes combined the salacious with the utilitarian, producing helpful devices like this one for the bones of the hand:

Sarah	Scaphoid
Looked at	Lunate
Tom's	Triquetrum
Powerful	Pisiform
Torso,	Trapezium
Getting	Groove of Trapezium
Titillated,	Trapezoid
Cerebrating	Capitate
Heavily:	Hamate
Mesmerizing!	Metacarpals

Sometimes, however, mnemonics and the V-2 Rocket were not enough. Picture yourself in this scenario:

It's 0700 Monday morning. You've been up for the last forty-eight hours on your emergency room rotation as a part of your internship at Anytown's Big County Hospital. Twelve of you, men and women, are packed into a tiny conference room without enough chairs. Some of your compadres are leaning against the walls, some are hiked up onto window sills. Each of you, in filthy, sweaty scrubs, smells like the Newark city dump—no time for showers in the recent past.

After meager rations of very strong coffee in plastic cups and very stale doughnuts in paper towels, an impeccably dressed attending surgeon—slightly graying, mustachioed, and much feared—enters. In his horn-rim glasses and long white coat, he takes a seat reserved for him. Without a preliminary word he says:

"Dr. Sawyer?" The room falls deathly quiet. The lion roaming the Serengeti has picked his lame gazelle.

"Yessir?" answers an exhausted intern.

"He's lying on the trauma table in the E.R. The ambulance crew has just stepped aside. He has one 18-gauge antecubital IV in his left arm wide open with lactated Ringers' solution. He is blue. What do you do?"

"I'd begin CPR," says Sawyer confidently.

"Excuse me. You'd do what?"

Again, with slightly less *savoir faire*: "I'd begin CPR."

"Don't you think you ought to check and see if he's breathing on his own before you decide to do it for him?"

"Well, yeah, I mean, sure. Check for respiration and if there is none, begin CPR."

"Hold it." The professor again. "Aren't we forgetting another tiny little detail, Doctor? Perhaps you're interested in his pulse. You remember, cardiac function? The 'C' part in 'CPR?'"

Now every intern knows the basics of CPR. The unsuspecting gazelle expected questions along the line of "How many milligrams of bretylium per kilo do you give in ventricular fibrillation after lidocaine, epinephrine and Isuprel have failed?" By now everyone in the room

23

knows what kind of morning it's going to be. This will not be fair pimping. This will be a bloody, ugly affair.

"O.K.! After I check for the absence of pulse, I begin CPR." Dr. Sawyer sounds somewhat exasperated.

"Oh, so tell me, Doctor, you don't think the pulse is all that critical to ascertain?" The sarcasm drips from the surgeon like mucous from the nose of a two-year-old.

"Yes sir, I think it's important." Sawyer's voice is losing its snap. The gazelle is tiring.

"Well, let's assume you're awake enough, Dr. Sawyer, to initiate CPR, start a central line, get the patient intubated, send off some blood gases, put some EKG leads on and get a pattern. What you see is the old QRST (normal heart wave patterns) lookin' just fine, but your patient has no pressure and isn't breathing. What are we dealing with?"

Well, every intern there knows the answer. EMD, electro-mechanical dissociation. But the gazelle on the fringe of the herd is beginning to panic now. He can feel the lion's hot breath on his hindquarters and he knows it's hopeless. His only hope lies in the rest of the herd drawing the lion's attention.

Not very damn likely. We've seen what kind of a morning this is. This is not a learning morning in the conventional sense. This is a learn-just-exactly-how-low-a-form-of-life-the-intern-is morning. Which means that jumping in with the answer will indeed turn the big cat's attention momentarily, just long enough for him to rip out your throat before returning to finish off the original quarry.

"I think it's that disassociated thing... sir." Dr. Sawyer's breathing is becoming labored.

The surgeon looks around the room. Suddenly, those plastic cups of cooling coffee seem worthy of intense study. Everyone manages to be looking elsewhere at the critical millisecond of visual intercept. The surgeon is disgusted.

"'That disassociated thing,' Doctor? What thing is that exactly?" the surgeon asks with a derogatory smirk.

"I guess it's where the electrical signal is present in the heart, but for whatever reason the pump can't supply a pressure?" Dr. Sawyer looks up fleetingly. Could the big cat's attention be turned elsewhere with a partially correct response? Not a chance.

"How do you help the man, Doctor?"

"I'd give him calcium chloride, epinephrine and start a dopa drip?" The panicked gazelle turning to fight? Does he think that he can dodge the onrushing, tightly wound bundle of pure muscular hellcat?

"Well, Dr. Sawyer, you do that. Nothing happens. Nothing. You're killing him—you know that, don't you? Every second is precious and you're standing around pumping him full of medicines that don't work while he dies. Are you gonna tell his family you were just too sleepy to think of the right approach? Are you?"

Only the rattle of the anemic air conditioner can be heard in the room. A few people shuffle to change position. Jesus! How long can this go on?

"No, ah, sir." The big buck is on his side now. Froth bubbles from his mouth. His dusty coat is turned muddy by the sweat. He furiously throws his head in the air one last time before the crushing jaws close around his neck.

"I'd do a paracentesis. Yeah, that's what I'd do. I'd take an 18-gauge spinal needle, insert it under the sternum to the left and aim upwards until I aspirated the pericardial fluid causing his tamponade!"

"And what is tamponade, Dr. Sawyer?"

"Well, the fluid trapped in the sac around the heart. The fluid compresses the heart and makes it an ineffective pump."

"So you'd put a needle in it and drain it?"

"Uh, yes sir."

"Oh, that would be excellent, Dr. Sawyer. Excellent. Then you wouldn't be guilty of incompetence. I'd say you'd be guilty of murder. Murder by pro-active stupidity. Remember when you were supposed to have intubated your patient? You were supposed to listen for breath sounds, remember? You wouldn't have heard them on the right while breathing for him with the ambu bag. Why not?"

"You're down a main stem bronchus?" says a new voice from the back. The lion never shifts his gaze from the original prey.

"You people amaze me. First of all, it's the right main stem bronchus that gets intubated accidentally, so that's obviously not the case here. Why don't we have breath sounds, Dr. Sawyer?"

"I... I... don't know." The razor sharp teeth sink through the loose hide over the windpipe, then rip a huge hunk out of the carcass.

"Ever heard of a tension pneumothorax, people? All this poor bastard needed was for this summa cum laude desk jockey here to put a 16-gauge needle in his right chest, bleed off the air in the pleural cavity, kick start him with a little epi if needed, and then place the chest tube. Well, Dr. Sawyer, it's only 0723 on a Monday and you've already killed somebody. How does it feel?"

Dr. Sawyer looks steadily at the floor. His eyes are glistening, his face frozen with humiliation and fury. He doesn't answer as the herd moves on, the surgeon now launching into a didactic covering acid-base balance and calculation of base deficit.

The prey lay in its own gore, flies gathering as the sun approached its zenith. This herd animal learned the hard way that the only protection from this kind of ferocious assault, the worst kind of pimping, was to be sure you knew all, and I mean *all*, the damn answers.

" Is My Tool All Right? "

PHYSICIANS DEAL WITH SOME HORRIBLE things, including the damage one angry person can do to another in a society where handguns are rampant. I've often wondered why the movies don't show what it's really like after someone has been shot. I don't mean the gore; there's more than enough of that. But they don't often show the agony, the writhing, or the abject terror.

In becoming a physician, I was exposed for the first time to some of these horrors. Up close, you learn that the body is all too easily destroyed. But you also learn that the body and the mind are inextricably entwined. Even in the bloody ruins of a gunshot victim's body, the human feelings that give him his identity live on. And regardless of the circumstances that brought this person to these last moments of pain and terror, he can be helped with a kind word—even if it stretches the truth.

Part of the physician's task involves recognizing the patient as a human being. That means more than merely remembering that your patients have feelings. It also means seeing all your patients as equally deserving of your best efforts to ease their suffering.

I was working again as a volunteer in the emergency room of the county hospital. It was about one o'clock on a Saturday morning. This was remarkable only in that Basic Science final exams were beginning on Monday and I didn't *have* to be in the E.R. But I wanted to be there. After all, the patients were the point, not the textbooks. We wanted to be where the action was. We wanted to do the "doctor thing" as soon as possible. Saturday night was the usual meeting of the "Knife and Gun Club." The Mexican gangs mostly used knives, probably for both cultural as well as financial reasons.

27

The blacks, on the other hand, used guns exclusively.

Well, if you have ever played "Rock, Paper, Scissors," you know that guns beat knives almost every time.

In any event, I was lying across the chest of a particularly exercised black male about twenty years old. I was one of several people trying to keep him on the trauma table while the nurses cut away his jeans to assess the damage he had suffered while exchanging fire with police. My immediate assumption, being an upper-middle-class white boy, was that he must have screwed up big time. The S.O.B. probably deserved whatever he got.

He was thrashing about, foaming at the mouth, jerking his head back and forth and screaming, "My tool, my tool, I gotta know, is my tool all right?"

It was a wonder he could speak at all. The right side of his face was gone, just flat-out gone. I remember as clearly as if it were yesterday that I could see all the way down his throat through a hole the size of a softball where his right cheek and jaw should have been. How could he even swallow his own blood and saliva, much less articulate those words? I didn't have a clue what his "tool" was or why he was so upset about that when half his face was gone.

Then the nurses got his pants off, and in turning my head to keep his spittle from my face, I saw why he was disturbed. Most of his upper left thigh was unrecognizable. But even more horrifying than the bloody wreck of his leg was the fact that only shreds of his scrotum and penis remained. As the blood poured from his groin and face and neck, his struggles became weaker. His shouting turned to moaning.

I knew he had been in a fight with the cops, but as he was dying in front of me, I couldn't help thinking what it must be like for him. I was twenty-two. I knew my "tool" certainly played a big part in my future, even if its current role was somewhat diminished by time constraints. Was it really so absurd that he should be more worried about his manhood than the ragged shreds of a face he had left?

I was still lying across his chest. As he weakened I leaned over and shouted in his ear, "It's all right, man.

Your tool is totally cool. Shotgun just caught your upper leg is all. You hear me, man? You're okay!"

He grabbed my shoulder with his right arm. His face, or what remained of it, was about six inches from mine. "Thanks, man, thanks a lot."

Those were his last words. He died right there. I got the hell out of the way and the people who knew what they were doing coded him for a while, but they gave up after about five minutes.

It turned out he was shot while robbing a liquor store. He'd killed an eighteen-year-old Vietnamese girl shortly after the police arrived on the scene. People around the trauma room got a laugh out of his concern for his genitals. Some made comments about how you'd expect that from one of the brothers.

Then an unexpected thing happened to me. I found myself furious with the people making fun of him. I was too young and naive to recognize their defense mechanisms for dealing with this horror, but I knew one thing: this poor bastard shouldn't have died at twenty, no matter what he'd done.

Many years later my father gave me a piece of paper he'd carried in his wallet for fifty-seven years. It was titled the "Sanibel Success Story."

> Success is the word for which there could be a thousand definitions. A great many people equate success with money.
>
> The fact is that there are millions of affluent failures and an equal number of successes who have nothing in the bank.
>
> One definition of success is to win the respect of intelligent persons and the affection of children, to earn the approval of honest critics and endure the betrayal of false friends.
>
> To appreciate beauty, to find the best in others, and to have accomplished a rescued soul.
>
> To have played and lived with enthusiasm and seen with exultation, to know that even one life has breathed easier because you have lived.
>
> This is to have succeeded.

These thoughts which my father valued so highly remind me of this story. This man deserved my help, no matter his color, his creed, his station, or his actions. I feel sorry for the girl he killed, but I have no regrets about what I said to him or did for him.

If for one brief moment before he died, this man breathed easier because of me, then that was successful medicine.

ORALS

NOW HERE IS A SADISTIC CONCEPT worthy of Torquemada himself. The Spanish Inquisition was no more adept at torture than modern-day academic oral examiners. This is the ultimate "rite of passage," the final "portal" through which many specialists must pass, which is why I include it in this section despite the fact that orals come two years after residency. Just the word "Orals" strikes fear and loathing into the hearts of those who have survived to practice medicine in the real world.

Orals are roughly comparable to the thesis defense for a Ph.D., but the consequences of failure are not the same. Failure on the oral exams in obstetrics and gynecology means not only humiliation for you and your residency program, but nowadays may also mean loss of the right to apply for hospital privileges, alteration of referral status for managed health-care plans, reduced reimbursement from those insurers that will still recognize you as a provider—in short, the end of the dream for which you have worked over the last ten grueling years.

Now remember, we're talking about abject terror here. We are not talking about nervousness. We are not talking about apprehension. We are not talking about a little anxiety. We're talking about finding Edgar Allen Poe's telltale heart on the pillow next to you after you switch on the light at three in the morning to investigate a noise in the house.

Remember also that we are talking about a very select subset of the world's population—a group of men and women who have already been tested more than the average person would be in ten lifetimes. These people already have their medical degrees. They have already completed at least eight years of pimping and been under fire in the trenches for the last four years. These people are not marshmallows. Most have just completed their

31

first two years in practice and just before that, their tours as chief residents. By this point they are much more accustomed to being the interrogator than the interrogee.

The torture really begins long before you arrive in the dungeon. The American Board of Obstetrics, Gynecology, and Infertility requires that the physician keep a detailed case list of every delivery and operation in the year before the exam. This list must include evidence of adequate exposure to all types of clinical situations. If either the form or content of the list, submitted four months prior to the exam, is deemed inadequate by some unseen god, you may be refused permission to sit for the exam until the following year. Once you receive notification of acceptance of your case list, family emergencies, deathly illnesses, floods, earthquakes, nuclear war are all unacceptable excuses for not appearing in the assigned city at the assigned time.

In my case the assigned city was Chicago. The assigned time was smack dab in the dead of winter. Cold? A bit. Howling gales. Tribes of Eskimos muklukking from one igloo to the next. You know what it feels like to fall through a sea lion's breathing hole into the Arctic sea? That is Chicago in the winter.

As I entered the lobby of the modern high-rise hotel where the orals were to take place, I ran into only one person I knew from Dallas. She had taken her test the day before and was now preparing to leave for the airport. Absolute piece of cake, she exclaimed. Examiners were pussycats. Don't worry about it!

My extensive test-taking experience told me that this was an extremely dismal sign. The implication was clear: the exam was a total bitch. So bad, in fact, that this relatively bright young doctor didn't even realize when she'd been wasted! Oh God! Now I was really worried.

The exam is in three parts: (a) microscope slides, (b) Kodachrome slides, (c) case-list review. The examiners can ask any question they deem appropriate related to the slide or Kodachromes in front of you or to a case chosen from your list.

Now only a truly demented mind could come up with some of these questions and claim they were related to what we had studied. Imagine that the slide concerns the *Titanic*. You have memorized dates, the number of decks, people, lifeboats, survivors, the name of the captain of the *Carpathia*, etc., etc. And here comes the question: "In the cold waters of the North Atlantic, what type of shark are you most likely to encounter?" Arggh.

My first two examiners were men. They asked relatively direct questions about the microscope slides and the Kodachromes. True, there were some photos of young men/ladies with ambiguous sexual characteristics, and no one could talk intelligently about them without a review of the appropriate genetics and biochemical pathways immediately before the exam. But there were only a few like that, and I was beginning to feel after the first two hours that I might never be pumping gas at a Texaco.

Then it happened. I entered another hotel room for my case-list review to find a very severe but attractive woman of about forty from Columbia University seated with a clipboard in her lap. She did not look up when I entered the room. I introduced myself, held out my hand, and asked her where she was from. Still not flattering me with even a glance, the examiner castrated me with this: "Have a seat. I don't really think this is the place for social pleasantries." Well, excuuuuuuuuuuuuse me!

The next forty-five minutes were unforgettable to say the least. This doctor dissected me like a cadaver. How, with a list of hundreds of cases, twenty examinees, and probably no time to read the list, could this hellcat zero in on the very few that I wished weren't on there! She used the laparoscopic cystectomy, which predated the procedure's popularity by about five years, to rip my lungs out. By the time the Kommandant was through with me, I was scheming about how I might eventually move from the pump to the cash register, then perhaps some day to assistant manager.

I don't know how I managed to check out, get a cab, and find the obscure airport concourse used for the puddle-jumper to Cedar Rapids, Iowa, where I would visit my old medical school roommate. While I waited for the plane at the gate, I called my wife back in Dallas. She deserved to know that, in light of the limited opportunities for advancement at the Texaco station, she would have to go back to work if the kids were going to go to private school.

I got her on the line and told her the test was fine right up until I met this incredible (while turning) BITCH (now seeing her waiting for the phone directly behind me) who destroyed any hope of a future for the two of us. Now I ask you: Chicago O'Hare, one of the biggest, busiest airports in the world, and who's out at gate 12,345 waiting for a puddle-jumper to Duluth? The catamount from Columbia. Any doubt about my flunking the orals vanished in her tight-lipped smile as she simultaneously recognized me and the reference to her own personality!

Did the examiners mail in their evaluations? Was there a vote among the three examiners preceded by discussion? Did the Inquisitor meet a fiery end just short of the runway in Duluth? Who knows? But some miracle did happen, because six weeks later I received notification by mail. I would not be applying at any local service stations. I had made it.

Now the good news! The American College of Obstetrics and Gynecology has decided that all physicians must be recertified (with orals) every ten years, or be removed from the college. Which graduating year did they pick as the first that would fall retroactively under these new rules? You guessed it. I'll be on the line again in 1998, but maybe this time I'll draw New Orleans. Houston. Bogotá! Anyplace but Chicago in the winter!

All of us have portals through which we must pass in our lifetime. Some are unavoidable: the death of parents, the ravages of age on our bodies, our children becoming independent and moving away. Some of them are by choice: college entrance exams, graduate school work, marriage (and, for some, divorce), having children. Oral exams for the physician are technically something he chooses to do, but definitely not something he would ever choose to do again. Living through them, however, teaches you priorities. After it's over, you realize that death was not actually imminent.

A wise person once said, "Don't ever confuse inconvenience with real problems." Isn't that the truth? Next time you think the world's crashing in around you, remember you could live in Bosnia or Rwanda or have some real problems.

As the neophyte physician achieves the self-awareness to recognize the portal process for what it is—i.e., a sequence of steps which must be taken, but which, if missed, do not represent the end of the world—he moves from *becoming* a doctor to actually *being* a doctor. While he may have a better perspective on his own career path, he is just beginning to understand that now, missed steps *can* mean the end of the world—for his patient. Part Two explores the grave responsibilities inherent in being a doctor.

"Words of compassion, skillfully
administered, are the oldest therapy
known to man."
—Louis Nizer

PART TWO

MEDICINE:
THE ART
OF COMPASSION

THE EXHAUSTING, MESMERIZING THRILL
of medical school gives way rapidly—
overnight really—to the exhausting new
responsibility of internship and residency, four
to six years during which the successful
physician will earn the moral and clinical
authority for medical decision-making. Then
he leaves residency and enters practice or
academics as a "real" doctor, someone whose
decisions are final and who holds the ultimate
responsibility for the patient's care.

At least that's how it was until fairly
recently. For most of my fifteen years in
medicine, I made diagnostic and therapeutic
choices with only these criteria in mind: what
would best serve the interests of my patient?
What would I do if this were my wife? As a
compassionate physician I suffer with my
patients, and I strive to alleviate their suffering
as if it were my own.

The following vignettes are drawn from a
time before health-care providers, when I truly
was a doctor.

CHANGE OF VENUE

MANY PEOPLE SUFFER from the illusion that American medicine is a clearly definable entity that is uniform from sea to shining sea. Having gone to medical school in one city, done my internship and residency in a second city, and settled in yet another for practice, I know that nothing could be further from the truth. Because medicine is an art and not a science, its practitioners vary widely from one part of the country to the next.

Having seen medicine practiced in different ways and in different places, the polished physician has the luxury of choosing from the best of the techniques learned, but there's often some culture shock along the way. For instance, if you ask a San Francisco scrub nurse for a "peon," she (1) looks as though she hasn't heard you, (2) says "say what?", or (3) in a moment of compassion, hands you the kelly and educates you as to the instrument's proper name. You could say the same for a "mosquito" and a "hemostat," a "schnit" and a "right angle," a "DeBakey" and a "fine atraumatic," an "Army-Navy" and an "s-retractor," a "malleable" and a "ribbon" or "fish."

But the differences run much deeper than medical terminology, extending to the people themselves. From one metropolitan area to another, the patients vary dramatically in their cultural makeup, as I learned in the early eighties when I served an internship in San Francisco, the city that put the "multi" in multicultural.

It was my first day at San Francisco General Hospital. I didn't even know where the bathrooms were yet. After an all too brief orientation, we interns were thrown to the wolves. About 6:00 p.m. I was doing my first delivery

39

as a real live M.D. I had delivered several hundred babies as a medical student at Jeff Davis Hospital in Houston, but this was my first as a doctor.

Cultural variation number one: In Houston in 1980, patients usually delivered in a very sterile, brightly lit room reminiscent of the standard operating room. In San Francisco, most patients delivered in a Holiday Inn–style room built into the hospital. It had everything but the magic fingers and the coin box.

O.K. I could adapt to this, no problem.

Next difference: In Houston, most women wanted an epidural. Pain was bad. In San Francisco, many women shunned epidurals. Pain was, if not bad, at least natural, and drugs (at least these drugs) were bad. Therefore, the typical patient in San Francisco could get very vocal as the pain increased. Naturally.

Finally, picture the soon-to-be doctor kneeling at the end of the Holiday Inn bed, bent over sideways with a wholly inadequate gooseneck lamp, trying desperately to visualize the torn "virginia" into which he was less than deftly placing sutures. The stirrups to which I had been accustomed were not in evidence, and the patient was forced to try to keep her legs bent at the knee and separated—all this while her pain was inadequately controlled with local anesthetic.

On this first day, I had forgotten that I was in a city where almost everyone wanted to deliver squatting in Golden Gate Park while chewing alfalfa sprouts. While Mom held her new baby, Dad slipped over to the delivery table behind me. He quietly removed his shirt. The labor nurse in the room took no notice of him whatsoever. Between stitches, I glanced in his direction and witnessed the first of many cultural revelations that were to broaden my horizons in the next four years. Dad reached in the plastic basin on the table and removed the placenta. Carefully rearranging the membranes so that the maternal side of the disc would be exposed, he proceeded to wipe the bloody organ all over his chest and face. Luckily, I was speechless.

When I regained my composure, I motioned to the R.N. to lean down in my direction.

"Does uh—does uh, everyone here do that?" I whispered. "And by the way, what is he doing?"

She gave a little chuckle as she went back to filling out the baby's arm bands. "He's from Marin, honey."

That was it. That was the total explanation. Marin, I was soon to learn, is the county immediately north of the Golden Gate Bridge. I began to sense that maybe we weren't in Kansas anymore.

Another first-day cultural variation. Scene: SFGH obstetrics clinic. I stood in the hall outside one of the gazillion draped cubicles that passed as exam rooms. All of the rooms were filled, largely with people for whom English was not even a second language.

As I dutifully waited for a nurse to accompany me in to examine the first patient, I noticed that I was the only intern standing in the hall. A three-hundred-pound black nurse noticed the same thing and ambled over. Ah, I thought, she's going to lend assistance to the greenhorn.

"What you waitin' on, honey?"

"I was just waiting for a nurse, thank you."

"What for? You need somebody to hold your hand?"

"Don't I need a chaperone in the room for an exam?"

She looked at me as though I were from not another state, but a distant planet.

"What you need to do, Doctor, is get your happy ass in there and see the patient!!"

"But... "

"The only butt I see out here is yours, and if you want to keep it outta the sling, you best get in there NOW!"

Needless to say, the gentilities of the Old South were not recognized with your average Vietnamese patient in the San Francisco county hospital. I quickly entered the room only to realize that the person I really needed was the interpreter, who arrived in due time.

Now let's jump ahead about four weeks. It was midnight at Moffitt Hospital. Labor & Delivery was on the fifteenth floor, overlooking the old Kezar Stadium, Golden Gate Park, and, in the distance, the lights on the Golden Gate Bridge. I had had a month to adapt to a very different style of delivery, usually in a birthing room. While I was initially less adept, I had adjusted and in

41

fact could at this point see considerable merit in unmedicated delivery in a nonsterile environment. As the midwives on staff taught me new tricks, I began to think I was pretty good at this and had seen the gamut of possible delivery styles.

My first educational experience that night came from a very attractive five-foot, ten-inch Swedish blonde having her first child. She and her husband had spent early labor in one of the well-appointed birthing rooms, listening to music and supporting each other with Lamaze technique. As it turned out, he was the Swedish consul to the United States in San Francisco.

When I went to check on her about 1:00 a.m., she was in transition, or about eight centimeters dilated. This is usually the most painful part of a first labor, and I did not anticipate her delivery for at least several hours. Immediately after I told them this, she first opened the front of her gown, then shed it completely. Her husband helped her to stand by the queen-size bed.

I must have looked surprised, because I remember her looking at me and asking if it was okay to be naked. Who was I to say no? She and her diplomat husband (who, thankfully, did not undress) proceeded to slow dance to Franz Schubert for the next two hours. It was actually remarkably beautiful. And definitely something I had not seen in Texas.

This couple taught me even more that night. After one and a half hours of pushing, during which she squatted and he supported her beneath the arms from behind, I delivered my first baby while lying flat on my back.

Not to be insensitive, but to imagine this, you have to have changed your own car's oil filter in the driveway. I might add that the anatomy of the pelvis is difficult to visualize normally, much less when you are upside down and backwards. Pulling the delivering shoulder "down" beneath the pubic bone takes on a whole new complexity when you're in that position.

But we accomplished it together, and another beautiful little blonde, blue-eyed Swedish girl entered the world. The special nature of the moment of birth overcame any of my concerns about awkward positioning or unexpected nudity.

As I noted earlier, it was not only the mechanics of medicine which I found markedly different in this new environment, but the mechanics of life in a culture whose reputation for tolerance was known worldwide.

After only several days at SFGH, I was exposed to yet another novel situation for the novice physician. My chief resident told me to work up an admission for a hysterectomy and bilateral oophorectomy to be performed the following day. After clinic ended that evening around seven, I called the operator and was told that this patient was on ward 3D in bed 321B. It wasn't a GYN floor, but occasionally we had overflow to other wards, so I thought nothing of it. At the nurses' station I grabbed the chart with "Harrison" on it, and after a brief knock on the door, cruised into a room occupied only by a large, well-muscled, thick-bearded truck-driver type. I excused myself with a simple "Sorry, wrong room" and didn't even wait for a response.

At the nurse's station, I asked an equally confused but slightly more annoyed clerk just where Miss Harrison had been deposited. She informed me that this was ward 3D. *Male* ward 3D. I mentioned to her that I was aware of that extremely useful fact, but was she aware that nevertheless, the computer felt 321B to be one "Terry Harrison's" room for the next several days? The clerk reached over the counter from her seated position, spun the chart around, and flipped open the plastic binder. Pointing to the stamp in the upper right corner of the first page, she looked at me and with her eyes only said, Whudduya think that says?

Without further discussion, I picked up the phone and asked the operator to page my chief. In a few minutes she called back.

"Say, Michelle, I'm on 3D looking for that woman you said needed the hyst tomorrow, and there don't seem to be any girl patients down here!"

"How do you know?" she responded.

"Excuse me?" I queried.

"Did you take a history, or even introduce yourself?"

"Did I introduce myself as a gynecologist to a 250-

pound guy with a beard? Well, no I didn't. Seemed like he might not like me interrupting his TV show."

"Well, *Doctor* (too much emphasis on the second word here), maybe if you talk to Terry you'll learn to broaden your horizons and alter your expectations at the same time!"

"You're the boss."

With considerable trepidation, I reentered Terry's room. Needless to say, "he" was not exactly the appropriate pronoun. Terry turned out to be a very pleasant transsexual. She/he had been taking male hormone for twenty years. While the sex-change operation from male to female is extremely well perfected, as I had witnessed in medical school, the female-to-male surgery is multistep, difficult, and, at that time, had poor cosmetic results. Terry, as fate would have it, was in fact a long-distance trucker. Despite gainful employment, she/he had never acquired adequate funds for this noninsured procedure. So she led the life of a man while avoiding sexual encounters that might be disillusioning, to say the least, to new partners.

And she/he was hampered by one more little inconvenience. Heavy, extremely painful menstrual periods can make long-distance trucking almost untenable for a woman; they make it worse for a man. When Terry was in the company of others, she/he would explain the sudden pains, the rushes to the bathroom, and the medications as the result of recurrent hernia pain.

Terry's operation was a success. It was still remarkably strange, however, to be operating on female internal genitalia while at the same time being able to look over the drape and see the endotracheal tube protruding from between a mustache and a beard.

Some interesting discussions followed with regard to hormone replacement. While many women fear loss of estrogen function, this one positively rejoiced. We pointed out the benefits of estrogen replacement such as lower risk of heart attack and avoidance of hot flashes and osteoporosis. The patient pointed out that he felt one giant step closer to being in the body he was wrongfully denied at birth by some undiscovered trick of hormonal biochemistry. No thanks, we could keep our estrogen replacement, and please, continue the testosterone injections during the recovery period.

Call me naive. I certainly was that! But I had begun to learn that we should treat all patients (read: people) with respect regardless of their outward appearance, just as we should regardless of their race.

San Francisco was indeed a change of venue. From the different medical instruments and techniques to a culture with totally different customs and new definitions of the "norm," it brought a shift of reference points far beyond what I had expected. But physicians are trained to adapt to new situations. If you can't adapt, you can't very well deal with that surgical problem that crops up when you least expect it.

SLEEP

ASK THE CHILDREN OF A PHYSICIAN where Dad (or Mom, as the case may be) was during their first dance recital, or their first T-ball game, or their sixteenth birthday party. "The hospital" will likely be the answer, because the only other possible response would be "asleep."

Call it drive, call it dedication, call it foolish, call it anything you want, but it's a fact: Physicians learn to subjugate the wants and needs of their families and friends and even themselves to those of their patients, who soon become the priority. The doctor may be due at home for dinner. The doctor may be a walking zombie after thirty-six hours without sleep. But diagnostic tests, IV placements, wound changes, record-keeping and family conferences must go on. Even before my children could tell time, they learned from their mother that "on time" didn't apply to Dad. If I swore I'd be home at six, it might well be nine, and that meant after bedtime—another twenty-four hours without seeing Papa.

Sleep! Now there is a completely radical concept! If you want to get any physician in a surgical subspecialty excited to the point where he makes your one-year-old, nonneutered Labrador, surrounded by bitches in heat, look tame by comparison, offer him three hours of uninterrupted sleep!

I do not exaggerate. I know from personal experience that the average intern/resident—despite days, weeks, or months of abstinence—can fall asleep while an attractive, libidinous, naked member of the opposite sex lies beside him.

This is no reflection on said physician's degree of interest in the act of coitus or other related modes of sexual interaction. It merely shows he's got his priorities in order. Those of us who have spent years running up (sleep) deficits that make Washington's deficits look like pocket change know that an opportunity to hit the pillow is not to be taken lightly.

Sleep. Ah, sleep! Sleep is not just a steak cooked to perfection. Sleep is not just that feeling of taking your ski boots off after six hours on the slopes. Sleep is not just removing your hard contacts after thirty-six hours of wear. Sleep is not even that muscle-convulsing, warm, wet wave of intense pleasure that accompanies the temporary insanity of orgasm.

No. Sleep is better! Much, much better!

When I was in college, my older brother (now a heart surgeon) used to tell me that he fell asleep in elevators. I scoffed, not being naive enough to believe his tales of woe. Right, I thought. And weren't you the one who had to trudge twelve miles to school in the snow with sixty pounds of books on your back because they didn't invent the school bus until three years later when I started kindergarten? Of course it turns out that I was the little brother of little faith. My turn to sleep by necessity in odd places finally arrived, and proved more dangerous to the public than Dover-dozing.

Now keep in mind that sleep deprivation is probably the most effective form of torture used in covert intelligence-gathering worldwide. Amnesty International has it listed in its official menu of things civilized governments don't do to people. We don't really know what sleep is, what it does, how it does it, or much about it at all, except that a certain amount of it is absolutely necessary for proper cognition, orientation, and memory, as well as all other identifiable emotional and physical functioning. Deprived of sleep long enough, you first become lethargic, then disoriented, then agitated, then quite frankly, stark, raving mad. Then you go see the patient in 321B.

The elevator nap, aka Dover-dozing, is really a safety mechanism. If it weren't for these quick encounters with the sandman, many of the nation's indigents would be under the knife of agitated, disoriented, just-short-of looney-tunes surgeons.

I have seen colleagues fall asleep while: eating, engaged in public speaking, riding in elevators, riding in ambulances, driving their cars, holding retractors, taking tests, reading X-rays, presenting a case to their pimper (See "Survival of the Fittest"), riding a bike, playing tennis, performing a pelvic exam, listening to a chest.

The remarkable thing is that I have yet to witness a major error that I felt was caused by sleep deprivation in the treatment of a patient. There is truly something remarkable about the old adrenal glands. If a patient is in deep kemshee (doo-doo), you can pull out all the stops instantly, awaken from a dead stupor, and do exactly what you were trained to do on *very* little sleep.

I'm sure the public views this as less than safe. Some states have naively instituted legislation to limit the number of hours in a shift for medical personnel in training at state-funded institutions. Hah! Like who are they kidding? When you've been up for the last thirty-eight hours but still have twenty-six patients to round on, one crisis working in the emergency room, another disaster in ICU, and your replacement just as bombed in the operating room, what are you supposed to do? Saunter over to the time clock and punch out? You work until the work is done and you're covered by the next schmuck. Period. End of story.

Let the legislators mosey on over to their nearest teaching hospital and take a look at who's delivering the care. Let them find a way to triple the M.D.s in county facilities nationwide (hello, tax hikes) and then talk to us about twelve-hour shifts and getting adequate sleep. When you're bleeding to death from the gunshot in your chest, a sleepy chest-cutter is better than no chest-cutter, right?

Now admittedly there's a lighter side to this issue. Every spouse of an intern can tell you of the lovely, romantic anniversary dinner that was spoon-fed to the barely conscious intern propped up on the couch. Said meal lasted only until said intern could be sleepwalked to the bedroom for the usual six-hour respite before the thirty-six-hour cycle began again.

I would awaken to the 5:30 a.m. alarm and have no memory of how I got home from the hospital, ate dinner, took off my clothes, and fell into bed. I couldn't begin to tell you the number of nights I wandered for blocks in the San Francisco fog, having no idea where I'd parked my Celica with its 120,000 miles the early morning of the day before.

But patients may rest assured: The danger began only after getting behind the wheel. If you have a patient's belly open, and she's bleeding to death from a ruptured ectopic, it doesn't matter when you slept last, baby, you are *wide awake.* But when you're in the familiar comfort of your driver's seat, essentially guiding the car on auto pilot through the same streets, the same turns, the same hills, the same lights, you can drift a bit.

Take the time I woke up with the bumper of my Celica on the boat hitch of the pickup in front of me. Take the time I rolled down one of those world-renowned San Francisco hills backwards in my one-week-old Jeep Cherokee and smashed into a nurse's one-day-old Mazda RX-7, completely filleting the hood from latch to windshield. Take the time the trolley car conductor had to shake me awake while my car straddled the rails, detaining angry tourists from their intended spending sprees. Take the time I drove the wrong way down the one-way street in Golden Gate Park, stopping just nose-to-nose with one of those funny cars with the flashing lights on top. Keep in mind, these are only some of *my* exploits. During any twenty-four-hour period, a big city public hospital may send one hundred to one hundred and fifty sleep-deprived interns and hundreds of slightly less sleep-deprived residents out on the highways. Besides those "Quiet" signs that surround hospitals, maybe we need "Caution: Interns Dozing!" as well.

After two years in San Francisco, my wife wanted more room than the eight-hundred-square-foot walk-up that we shared with our Siamese. I said, "Why on earth would you want to move? We just got here."

That's when, using her laptop computer, my wife demonstrated that I had in fact actually "lived" in the apartment five-fold less time than she had, or the equivalent of four and one-half months. No wonder I felt like we'd just arrived. We further calculated that I spent 90 percent of my time in that apartment unconscious, so that I remembered being there the equivalent of only thirteen and a half days! It was a moot point anyway. On $13,000 a year in the most expensive city in America, Russian Hill wasn't exactly beckoning.

So sleep. Enjoy it. Revel in it. Wrap it around you like a down comforter in winter, splash in it like a cool running stream in summer. But don't ever take it for granted. I guarantee your doctor doesn't.

GOOD GRIEF

IT COMES IN MANY FORMS, GRIEF. It can be a silence, a contemplation of something once possessed but lost long ago. Or it can be more immediate. Then it comes in waves, rolling, relentless, inescapable. It can be so oppressive that it actually takes on physical qualities. Thick, seemingly impenetrable, sometimes even suffocating.

Everyone has things to mourn in their lives. We all grieve at the passing of loved ones. But the commonality lies only with expected deaths. Most of us expect our grandparents to die before our parents, and our parents before our siblings or spouses, and ourselves before our children.

Physicians, in company with only the clergy and the undertaker, must deal not only with expected deaths, but also with those most horrible events for which the patient and her loved ones are completely unprepared. The most stressful event that a human being can experience is roundly agreed to be the loss of a child. It appears to matter little whether that child is one minute old, or seventy years old. The twenty-year-old mother of the term stillbirth may well understand the anguish of the ninety-year-old, the death of whose seventy-year-old son antedates her own.

It was at San Francisco General that I first witnessed the inconsolable sadness that comes from such a loss—and tasted the bitter dregs of abject failure as a doctor.

The young woman was eighteen, an indigent Laotian who presented with no prenatal care at thirty-four weeks Her extended family was with her. She had become sick several days before with vomiting, jaundice, diarrhea, progressive fatigue and disorientation, and finally incoherence. It was only then that her family rejected provincial attempts at therapy and called an ambulance.

Shortly after the young woman's arrival in labor and delivery, a sonogram revealed that the fetus had not survived the rapid onset of her mother's undiagnosed and untreated toxemia. The disease process had left the mother horribly swollen, hypertensive, close to coma, and with rapidly deteriorating liver and kidney function. She was, however, in labor at eight centimeters and would deliver soon.

Largely through hand gestures, we let the family know the fetus had died. As for the girl, the only Lao interpreters on staff were not of her Mien mountain area and knew little of her dialect. So, minutes after her arrival, knowing nothing of her infant's fate, she began bearing down with the strain of impending delivery recognizable worldwide. She was rushed on a gurney to a delivery/OR and placed on the table in stirrups.

At that time, families were not allowed in the delivery rooms, and I remember the nurses and the interpreter physically restraining the woman's young husband and distraught parents. From where I sat at the foot of the table, I could see them sobbing and shouting intermittently through the glass wall that divided the operating room from the rest of labor and delivery.

The pain of the delivery had momentarily brought the girl to full consciousness, and she struggled against the anesthesiologist's attempts to mask her with some nitrous oxide. Despite her inability to understand us or cooperate, the delivery itself was uncomplicated. When she saw her bloated, meconium- (dark green) stained, lifeless child, she began to roll her head back and forth and moan in an indescribable wail.

I sewed her perineum rapidly and was just about finished when the anesthesiologist noted a further loss of orientation and a froth bubbling from her mouth. Within seconds the patient's wailing was replaced by a sickening gurgle, then stillness. We called a code at that point and immediately began CPR while she was intubated. I'll never forget the fluid that jetted out the endotracheal tube with each chest compression. She literally had drowned in her own secretions as the capillaries of her lungs gave in to the effects of the amniotic fluid embolus that was robbing her of life beneath our hands and high-tech instruments.

She began to bleed vaginally, gushing like a bathtub faucet. During the next two hours, with at least twelve team members in the room, she received over thirty units of blood, twenty liters of saline, sixty units of fresh frozen plasma, and was cardioverted five times. Yet nothing could halt the inexorable doom set in motion by this rare embolic process. When we finally called a stop to it, the floor was ankle deep in body fluids.

By the time she was declared dead, a Mien Laotian sanitation worker had been summoned from his home to act as interpreter. The family simply could not believe that their loved one was gone, at first. After steadfastly refusing to accept our account of her death, they insisted on seeing her before transfer to the morgue. She was still in that God-awful room with her blood on the floor and the endotracheal tube in her mouth, further distorting the features already altered by bloating and discoloration. I shall never forget her father sinking to his knees, rolling on the floor, and beating the blood-soaked linoleum with both clenched fists. His moan sounded exactly the same as the one his daughter had delivered hours before at first sight of her dead child. Nearly everyone in the room was crying.

All of us interns and junior residents learned a lot in the ensuing five days as the case was researched and presented at conference. We learned, when the lab work came back, of her preeclampsia (toxemia), the ensuing abruption (placental separation), and fetal death, the coagulation abnormalities brought on by that process combined with prolonged retained dead fetus, combined with liver failure, combined with the crowning blow of amniotic fluid embolus. But those of us who were there learned much more than the physiology.

Those of us who had never faced the death of a patient in our care will not forget that day. Mortality comes crashing home when you see the life of a teenager pumped out onto the floor.

I heard a message in the common moan of father and daughter, a message that has shaped me as a physician far more than the understanding of her disease process. That message has many layers, but certainly a central part of it is that what we do is very important to people. Oh, they may not say it much anymore, but people really do put their lives in doctors' hands, and the loss of any life brings home the gravity of our responsibility. I think all physicians get that portion of the message.

There is another part of the message which most, but not all, physicians come to understand: Our patients expect more than medical expertise and judgment. They expect us to be healers of both body and spirit. And yet, too great an emotional investment in the spiritual renewal of a devastated patient or loved one can rapidly destroy a practicing physician.

It is a tightrope between callous aloofness on the one side and complete surrender to despair on the other that the physician must walk. In recent months, one of my partners or I had to tell a twenty-seven-year-old just back from her honeymoon that she had breast cancer; remove the cancerous kidney of a woman twenty-eight weeks pregnant with twins who thought she would never live to see their second birthdays; console the mother of an eight-week-old girl who died of SIDS; help the mother of a two-year-old who had been crushed beneath a garage door operated by her five-year-old; comfort the mother of a two-year-old who had pulled over his dresser drawers at nap, suffocating himself; support a thirty-seven-year-old woman just after discovering on ultrasound that, after eight years of infertility and subsequent successful in vitro fertilization, her twelve week fetus was dead; and meet repeatedly with parents whose baby had died moments after birth of meconium aspiration while the grandparents and great-grandparents looked on in the birthing room.

Such events, while rare in the lives of most people, are almost daily occurrences for the physician. Many physicians become emotionally involved in the care of their patients, and rightly so. Many times I have cried with a patient or her family because I truly shared in their anguish. Certainly there are those who are trained specifically in dealing with grief—psychologists, social workers, and chaplains. But the family physician of long standing can help, perhaps more than anyone else, with healthy grief counseling.

But who will heal the healer? There is always the next patient, and that patient also wants and deserves the doctor's emotional investment. Moments after discussing the probability of an ovarian cancer with a woman who has just seen her own mass on the sonogram screen, the doctor must walk to the next room and share the joy of the long-term infertility patient who sees her eight-millimeter-sized fetus for the first time!

It takes tremendous energy to alter one's demeanor rapidly and repeatedly, day in and day out, changing your mood to mirror the patient's. A few physicians cope by withdrawing emotionally. So far that hasn't happened to me, and I hope it never does. Feeling too much may mean a slight loss of objectivity, but the human interaction fostered by empathy outweighs any inefficiency.

Recently my four-year-old son came into the bedroom one afternoon I had off. I had just finished talking to my minister about the death of a newborn. Although I knew I had not been responsible, I was distraught over the grief and anger of the patient's family. I had been sobbing to the extent that, when Andy saw my face, he started crying too. Later he told a teacher at my wife's Bible study fellowship that his daddy had cried because a baby had died. He was told that it was good his daddy could cry over things like that, and Andy seemed satisfied.

Well, overall, I think the teacher was correct. It is good that a physician can cry like that. But it didn't feel good. Not at all.

So the next time a physician strikes you as cold or unfeeling, think about what he might have had to tell the patient right before you. Some of us just shift gears a little faster than others. We only hope that rapid gear-shifting won't leave the mechanism stripped, or be replaced with a "managed-care automatic transmission," whereby the doctor makes a cash transaction with the "customer" and the patient ceases to exist.

The degree to which the doctor can truly participate in the spiritual healing of his patient cannot help but be linked to the longevity of their relationship. The revelation of intimacies, the counselling through difficult times, and the gradual relaxation of defenses between two people that occurs with the development of trust defines the doctor-patient relationship. As we shall see, the health-care provider at your health maintenance organization (with whom you have spoken once) may not be able to deal with whatever grief you might face in quite the same manner as your doctor could do.

I write this chapter in the evening of a particularly harrowing day. After four days out of town, I returned to find that one of my long-term infertility patients had lost her pregnancy at twenty-two weeks due to unexpected rupture of membranes and ensuing infection and labor. My partners had done all the right things. They had behaved professionally and compassionately. They had explained everything to the best of their ability. Still, this morning, the day after her loss, she burst into tears and held open her arms when I walked into her room.

I sat on her bed and held her in my arms for several moments until her sobs subsided. Her husband had his hand on my shoulder throughout, and didn't hide his own tears. Despite a packed schedule, I spent the next forty-five minutes talking with the two of them. We covered ground I knew my partners had already covered, but they wanted to hear it from me. We discussed the emotions she would experience, from denial to anger to bewilderment to fear and finally to resolution. We talked about the future. We talked about whatever needed talking about. Despite the guilt I always feel at not being there for the patient when a crisis occurs, she said as I left, "Thank you for being here. You don't know what a difference it makes."

I do know what a difference it makes, to me and to the patient. I know that without the ability to touch a patient and relieve her suffering there would be no reason to do what I do for a living. And even though there may be many doctors who don't take advantage of these windows of opportunity to truly heal, many of us do. I don't want you to lose the chance to have a doctor who really knows and cares for you, in exchange for a doctor who has only seen you once, or never seen you at all, and who, after all, gets off at five.

"Let 'Em
See You Sweat"

DOCTORS ARE IN NO WAY INFALLIBLE. In
fact, our mistakes may be more evident than
most professionals', because of the nature of
our work. If in a frenzied moment he makes a
flawed judgment, the good doctor recognizes
the error, makes appropriate changes, and
moves on.

But you can't learn from mistakes if you
won't acknowledge them. The patient must
view the doctor as even-keeled, as William
Osler counseled, but the med-school
admonition, "Never let them see you sweat,"
is bad advice for the doctor-patient
relationship. A patient cannot trust a physician
who perceives himself as infallible, because
inevitably the doctor will prove that he is
not—perhaps at the patient's expense.

In *Kindergarten Cop*, the harried Arnold Schwarzenneger
gets a splitting headache from dealing with his pint-sized
charges. When his partner offers her own diagnosis and
insists that the pain might have a more ominous origin,
Arnold lays down the law: "EETS NOTTA TUMOOR!"

No book focusing on the making of a surgeon
(gynecologic, that is,) could fail to include the well-meant
misdiagnoses of nongynecologists when it comes to the
female reproductive organs. Let's look first at the "It's
not a tumor!" category.

I was awakened one night at around three-thirty while
on call as a junior resident at San Francisco General
Hospital. This was unusual only in that I was actually
asleep and miraculously had been for over forty-five
minutes. The three interns covering labor and delivery
and the emergency room were evidently in total control
or, alternatively, had nothing to do.

In any event, the page was from a senior internal

medicine resident who was screening intern presentations in the ER. He listened to the case of a Laotian woman who was writhing in pain, hands clutching her abdomen, and who apparently had a large pelvic-abdominal tumor. As is often the case with indigent, non-English-speaking Asian patients, she evidently had not recently been a supplicant at this shrine of Western Medicine. It's not uncommon for such patients to arrive in the emergency room with advanced malignancies in a crisis stage.

The internal medicine resident, diligent fellow that he was, had personally examined the patient and confirmed the intern's findings. There was in fact a large, rock-hard pelvic mass at the apex of the vagina which seemed to extend in an irregular configuration all the way to the sternum. There was a small amount of blood from the opening of the cervix on speculum exam, but the upper vagina otherwise looked normal to visual inspection.

When I arrived in the tiny curtained space in the packed emergency ward, I discovered what can only be described as bedlam. The patient, who appeared to be about seventeen years old, was sweating heavily, flushed, and agitated. There was a woman by the head of the bed in tears, with her arms and upper body thrown across the thrashing patient's chest. Furthermore, the tiny space contained the ER intern, a nurse, and two security men restraining the presumed father, who was babbling unintelligibly and gesticulating wildly with alternating arms as he yanked away each arm in turn from those trying to restrain him. He seemed to be hurling most of his Laotian invective at our hapless internal medicine resident. In this quiet, calm group of professionals they needed me?

Anybody appraising this situation could tell one thing immediately: there were just too many people screaming in this tiny space. I asked security to remove the distraught gentleman and asked the two other physicians to give me a moment alone with the patient. When the noise level was down to only the patient's groans and the mother's sobs, I asked one of the only things I know how to say in French: "When was your last period?"

Well, the question seemed to silence the mother. The

teenager looked up and said, "I don't know," which was about the only other thing I know in French. With the nurse's help, the patient allowed a brief bimanual pelvic exam to confirm the impending birth. Quite remarkably, after we communicated this upcoming event with some unmistakable international sign language, the mother began once again to sob and wail and the daughter to thrash and groan.

The other physicians were of course mortified at my findings, almost to the point of self-vaporization. Once a translator had been obtained, however, it became clear that only the patient herself suspected her actual diagnosis. The parents practiced the Eastern version of Western denial, believing steadfastly that this occurrence was not possible since their daughter had not yet enjoyed sexual congress. I was tempted to tell the translator that she may not have enjoyed it, but she'd definitely had it. I remembered my professional code of conduct at the last instant.

This is not as outrageous as it seems. Doctors are no more omniscient than they are infallible, and many a patient has intentionally or inadvertently misled those attempting to care for her. In this case, denial was so manifest that this Laotian family either really didn't know what was happening or considered it so unlikely that they denied the logical findings of their own senses. Thanks to their demeanor on arrival and thereafter, the intern was sucked in completely.

And who can blame him? All doctors have seen people with large, previously undiagnosed cancers. The family's agitation told the unfortunate intern that something extremely grave must be happening here and made it easy for him to overlook the patient's youth, the fact that her pain came in waves, and even that on exam this mass felt just like a baby was supposed to feel! The resident, listening to hundreds of case presentations that evening, had hurried his exam and simply bought what the intern had told him.

Now, before you think that I'm libeling another specialty, consider the following scenario. Two years before I came to SFGH, there was a case that will live in infamy, a case that the responsible doctor involved will carry like a millstone around his neck forever.

Once again it is 3:00 a.m., a favorite time for disasters in medicine. The chief OB resident is called to labor and delivery for a screaming, morbidly obese woman who is bleeding vaginally and clutching her generous abdomen.

"The baby! The baby!" she shrieks. "Oh my God! My God! The baby's coming RIGHT NOW!"

Well, that kind of talk is bound to get attention. The nurses had listened for fetal heart tones and reported them as 70 (normal 120–160). Without immediate intervention, the fetus might die or be severely damaged. The senior resident had to make the call as the patient was rushed on a gurney to labor and delivery. He was waiting to examine her as she was wheeled in from the elevator. His bimanual exam revealed a single footling breech, and the patient was taken around the corner to the OR where she was "crashed" (put rapidly to sleep) and sliced open vertically for a cesarean section.

Everything went well with the surgery. The patient made a nice recovery. The hang-up was that she hadn't been pregnant—ever.

How is this possible, you ask? Were these doctors just careless or complete idiots? The answer, of course, is that they were neither. They were human. Patient's heart is pounding—so is yours. Patient's afraid her baby's going to die—so are you.

The woman was not pregnant. She was, however, quite sick. She suffered from pseudocyesis, a very real psychiatric diagnosis in which a schizophrenic patient, very convincingly, I might add, believes herself to be pregnant. The disorder presumably derives from a fervent desire to have a child in the face of some reason why this cannot be the case at the time—sterility, no sex partner, etc.

The senior resident, not unlike our intern in the ER, not unlike the nurse who heard the patient's pulse and believed it to be a fetus's heart, was completely sucked in. He *knew* this lady was pregnant before he examined her. Thus, the tampon he felt during the pelvic exam quite naturally became a foot prolapsing through the cervix.

The patient, incidentally, was not angry in the least. She did, however, grieve the loss of her imaginary child, and only when she was admitted to the psych ward on the first floor was it discovered that she had been discharged one week before. Diagnosis? You guessed it! Pseudocyesis.

Maybe this debacle was a failing on the part of all the people who had cared for her. Maybe it was only a failing on the part of a choked medical records system. But it certainly demonstrates the fact that physicians and nurses are human and empathize with patients whether they want to or not. And it reminds us that separating rational thought from adrenaline-driven impulses is difficult to do.

Recently I had the privilege of observing in a sophisticated Boeing 767 virtual reality simulator. Practicing takeoff from O'Hare into a thunderstorm with downbursts, both of the experienced pilots killed us three times apiece. Even knowing what to expect, they made the same instinctive error repeatedly.

Why? Because they were forced to react quickly without opportunity for contemplation. Even in a simulator you could feel their fear like a palpable thing. In slow motion they would have realized that forcing the nose up while averting an aborted takeoff, crashed the tail section into the runway and destroyed the aircraft. The flight computer never erred on multiple trials in the same situation, but the flight computer knows nothing about fear.

We can all be led astray by our initial impressions and be further confused by the emotions of those around us. Learning to evaluate "just the facts, ma'am" is difficult but essential for all of us, whether doctor, lawyer, pilot, or Indian chief, if we want to make the right decisions. Don't get me wrong: There are many instances where the pilot can outperform the computer by virtue of his human qualities of judgment, perseverence, and experience. By the same token, as pointed out previously, the doctor who can empathize may better serve some patient needs by demonstrating his compassion, and thus his humanity.

Being a good doctor requires the cool, clockwork rationality of the flight computer—and more. While the pilot must recognize his own emotions and fears but *never* show them to the crew or passengers, the doctor must learn that his own emotions and fears are the same as his patients' and that occasionally revealing them can be beneficial to the doctor-patient relationship. Achieving the desired outcome while still remaining human requires both compassion and self-discipline. These virtues are learned not in the flight simulator of medical school, but in the cockpit, in the air, in real practice, with precious lives in your care. Every now and then, let 'em see you sweat. They won't trust you completely if you don't.

BEING PATIENT

"WALK A MILE IN MY SHOES." Or just walk to the bathroom dragging an IV and wondering if your behind is showing through that ridiculous hospital gown designed by La Voyeur. We doctors can intellectually acknowledge the fear, the uncertainty, the embarrassment, and most of all the helplessness of our patients, but being patients ourselves changes mere sympathy to empathy. Once we've been "the broken leg in 135" or "the gall bladder in 316," we cannot help but meet the next patient's needs better than we did before our own health crisis.

I had awakened with what I thought was the usual morning stiffness—a gift, as we all know, from the God of Approaching Forty. I intended to head for the shower, first making the obligatory stop at my top bureau drawer for the morning's 800mg ibuprofen. Unfortunately, as I attempted to stand beside the bed, an excruciating pain shot down the back of my left leg to my heel.

As if that weren't bad enough, my foot suddenly began ignoring the important messages being sent earthward by areas of higher brain function. I had to drag it behind me, the perfect picture of the classic "foot drop" and a virtual tribute to Charles Laughton in *The Hunchback of Notre Dame*. Sitting, lying, squatting brought no relief to the intensifying sciatica.

I had previously experienced the complete paralysis of paraspinous muscle spasm, spending two scenic days in traction on the orthopedic floor at my very own hospital. On this occasion, however, the muscle spasm was mercifully absent. Consequently, I was able to drive to work, after a fashion, lying on my left side with the seat reclined, working both pedals with my good right foot. The pain down my buttock, thigh, and calf was excruciating. Phenomenally, I killed no one on the drive to the hospital.

Using all my worldly influence as a frequent and loyal referring physician, I was able to finagle a visit with the neurosurgeon—*two days* later. They might as well have told me they'd slip me in when the House of Representatives has a Republican majority!* Martyr that I am, I literally dragged myself through the next forty-eight hours, seeing patients but cancelling surgery left and right, and of course complaining bitterly every gimpy step of the way.

On the appointed day I spent the better part of the afternoon at the Southwest Imaging Center, a large facility that takes up the bottom two floors of one of the professional buildings on the hospital campus. When I arrived at the window wearing scrubs and white coat, I was strafed with the silent appraisal of the waiting room's septuagenarian and octogenarian occupants. There were no vacant seats, but this wasn't all bad since sitting was excruciating. I leaned against a column and tried to concentrate on a copy of *Preventive Health*, one of my personal favorites.

After less than three minutes a technician called out, "Dr. Thurston?" If looks could kill, I would have been vaporized in an instant. Fifteen pairs of tired but intense eyes, set in careworn faces, bored through my head with laserlike intensity. I felt like an ax murderer just released on a technicality. (Thankfully, as it turned out, I wasn't receiving special treatment. The technician told me that none of the other patients were waiting for the MRI machine.)

The technician turned me over to a late fiftyish schoolmarm of a nurse who directed me to a small change room and instructed me to undress completely, put on the gown, then sit on the bench outside the change room and wait.

I pulled the curtain, undressed, and fretted momentarily about where to leave my wallet. Finally, I just put it in my front pants pocket with the keys, somehow reassured that no thief would ever look farther than the right hip pocket for a wallet.

As I donned the threadbare hospital gown, open to the rear, I made the executive decision that "completely"

*Archaeological evidence that this was written before November 8, 1994 didn't mean removing my underwear. Feeling ridiculous, I threw open the curtain and prepared to lurch the short distance to the bench. A half-glass door immediately across the hallway opened and, with no schoolmarm in sight, out swept Christie Brinkley in a nurse's uniform. A very tight, curve-hugging nurse's uniform. She tossed her perfect, wavy blonde locks over her shoulder in that provocative way that little girls must learn to do in kindergarten. Her smile/giggle revealed a million jiggawatts of perfect pearly whites.

"Everything, Doctor. You'll need to take off everything, including your underwear. You're up, so I'll wait here for you." She shooed me back to the curtained cloister, arms out straight, hands bent down at the wrist, fingers flicking back and forth. My God, it was Marilyn Monroe in *The Seven-Year Itch*!

I retreated to the change room and for no earthly reason found that I regretted my dark socks, moderate pot belly, and love handles. I am perfectly happy in my marriage and cherish my wife above all else. Why should I care what Marilyn or Christie or whoever thinks about my socks? Right!

"Are you ready, Doctor? We've gotta move." As the 1992 *Sports Illustrated* Swimsuit Model of the Year helped me into the MRI scan room, I managed to grab hold of and pseudo-approximate the open rear of my flimsy, grossly inadequate gown. She positioned me on my back on the rock-hard, ice-cold table with my knees bent and supported by three pillows.

My embarrassment faded as I caught sight of the tubular tomb into which I would soon be propelled for the MRI. Believe me, the claustrophobic prospect of lying perfectly still, not to mention the throbbing agony down my backside, was adequate to eliminate any fleeting concerns I may have had over exposing my love handles to Vandela, Claudia Schiffer, or whoever.

As I contemplated the terror-eliciting potential of the scanner, Elle McPherson was putting a tourniquet on my arm. Yeow! That hurts when they twist off your arm hair! I *hate* needles. *Hate, hate, hate* needles. She deftly dug in an 18-gauge, (about the diameter of a sewer pipe) and warned about a possible "flushed" sensation as the contrast ran in. Liquid fire coursed through my veins as she positioned both my arms over my head. The table began to creep toward the black hole of the scanner a few maddening centimeters at a time. I closed my eyes and tried not to picture the inside of this sarcophagus.

It's incredible to me that man has the power to throw a ball accurately, hit one reliably, visually distinguish three millimeters at twenty feet, fly supersonic jet fighters, and play air hockey, but cannot control his own body's manifestations of anxiety. After about two and a half years of lying perfectly still, I began to get restless legs. You know, that sensation you get, usually at night, that you just *have to move!* After several stern admonishments from the disembodied voice over the intercom, I was able to force my thoughts away from movement to more pleasant topics, like what a mess my schedule was going to be after returning from surgical leave.

After another fourteen months, the scan was finished. I suffered the further indignity of trying to get to my feet essentially naked before the Athenian Goddess and being directed down the hall and to the left to the men's room. I was distinctly conscious of the cool draft on my rear, although I probably only imagined her gaze.

A few minutes later I returned and stepped up a step into the glassed-off reading room. The computer images were just coming up on the screen, and even a gynecologist could see a large hunk of lumbar disc material protruding into an area for which it was not intended.

"Big sucker, idn't it?" The tech queried before realizing it was I who looked over his shoulder.

"Oh, sorry, Doc," he said. "Guess that hurt, huh?"

"Yeah." I grimaced as I shuffled back toward the change room, ever-present right hand behind to ensure bottom modesty.

After about eight difficult minutes trying to get dressed while unable to bend over or use my left foot, I emerged once again. The perfectly proportioned and obviously healthy swimsuit model handed me my copy of the films after another wait of fifteen or twenty minutes. She gave me that perky little sand-and-surf smile and said she really hoped I'd be feeling better soon. I felt about eighty-seven years old, and my thoughts of her in a string bikini prancing effortlessly on the beach reinforced my geriatric self-image.

I found my way back to the front desk and finally reestablished contact with the schoolmarm. She directed me to the proper clerk, who finally found my paperwork only to tell me that there was nothing further I needed to do. I waited for a seventyish woman who obviously had more strength than I at the moment to open the office door, and I hobbled slowly down the corridor to the elevators.

In the neurosurgeon's waiting room it was *déjà vu*: same grumpy patients, same visual persecution when I was called back to an examining room after only a few moments. While I felt guilty, I was pleased because the pain was getting worse, not better. The nurse took some rudimentary information, laid the proffered films on the desktop, and told me the doctor would be right in.

I remember the room had an exam table that, in my debilitated state, was too high for me to get onto without a step stool. There was none in evidence. There was a small desk and phone, but no chair and no windows. I leaned against the exam table and studied the MRI images. It was probably only about twenty minutes later when I started to get annoyed. Couldn't they just pop in and give me a hint as to how long it would be? I decided to kill time by calling my office. If I was going to have disc surgery in the next day or two, it was time to start rescheduling the patients I wouldn't be seeing.

After several minutes on the phone, I made an abortive attempt to get up on the hard, leather exam table. The pain was unrelieved in any standing or sitting position, so finally I just lay on the floor. My trusty Seiko now told me we were going on one hour and fifteen minutes. Still no word from Nurse Ratchet. I rolled over, used the table to get to my feet, then opened the door a crack. She was sitting at a desk in a room across the hall eating a jelly donut and drinking coffee. She laughed with someone else in the room whom I couldn't see.

"Excuse me. Do you have any idea when he'll be here?" My exasperation was unmistakable.

"We'll let you know. Remember, you're an add-in. You know how that is, right?"

I knew how that was, right, but I also knew my nurses would be doing something to keep the patient more comfortable—offering a drink, a boost onto the table, or some help to the bathroom.

Dr. Hankins finally swept into the room just shy of 110 minutes after I had been deposited there. He looked up from his chart, shook my hand, and then helped me onto the exam table. I'm sure he was tied up in surgery, but he didn't mention it.

After I failed each part of the neurological exam, he gave the films a perfunctory review and then offered me two choices: I could live with it and hope it got better or operate on the disc. In light of the fact that I too was in a surgical subspecialty, working long hours bent over operating tables and generally abusing my back, he must have been aware that my current level of functioning would be woefully inadequate. I opted for the surgery.

It was scheduled for three days later. In the interim no amount of pain reliever, muscle relaxant, or massage seemed of much benefit. When my wife drove me to the hospital at 5:45 on D-day, it was still pitch black outside. We parked underground, and I hobbled to Admitting.

The first order of business there was to discuss "living wills" should I end up on life-support indefinitely. Well, my surgery was not a heart-lung transplant, and dying hadn't really crossed my mind. There's got to be a better way to greet the patient than this.

I met with the ubiquitous, too-short, threadbare, open-in-the-back hospital gown again shortly thereafter. My pastor came to visit and pray with me, further reinforcing my perception of approaching doom. As he was preparing to leave, a pretty young nurse (also ubiquitous) came in with an enema bag. After my initial shock and embarrassment, I remembered that after all this was an operation on my back, so I asked to see the doctor's orders. The enema order had not come from my neurosurgeon, but from one of my partners. Hardy har har.

Even riding on the gurney, watching the ceiling tiles flash by, was an unexpectedly uncomfortable experience. In medical school at Baylor we had been forced to "experience" being the patient by practicing on each other. We drew each other's blood, put down nasogastric tubes, placed Foley catheters, did rectal and pelvic exams, etc. But we never thought to whisk each other down a hall, flat on our backs on a gurney.

Well, I survived the operation. In fact, I even got to do it again exactly one year later. I had been holding two bottles of wine in my right hand—a Christmas gift from a patient—and my briefcase in my left. When it came time to retrieve my car keys, I carefully avoided bending to put down my briefcase. No, instead I did something much more stupid. I transferred the wine to the crook of my right arm and the briefcase to my right hand, then twisted around and reached into my right pocket with my free left hand. Brilliant! If someone else had been in the parking lot they could have heard the disc rupture. I screamed, fell to the floor, and got to do it all over again.

"Yuck," is the best way to express my experience as a patient. I don't think it was the pain, or the fear, or the embarrassment that made it awful. I think it was the helplessness. The patient is truly at the mercy of those who care for him or her. You become an object to which things are done. I believe it's around age two that we seek to become masters of our own environment. Loss of our autonomy at any age beyond that is at the least unpleasant, and at the worst terrifying.

There is no question in my mind that being the patient at some time or another is almost a necessity for developing into an empathic physician. In my personal case, however, I will strive to keep those instances to a bare minimum!

ON CALL

LIKE THE PERENNIAL LACK OF SLEEP, being "on call" shapes the life of the primary care physician or surgeon. Any moment of our lives can be (and often is) disrupted by that electronic umbilical cord, the beeper. While this is obviously detrimental to family life, the "call" phenomenon also focuses a doctor's entire life on medicine. Whether good or bad on balance, life on call is an inescapable fact for those who deal with problems that never seem to arise on schedule.

Certainly everyone has been required to "stand by" for some reason or other during their lives. Perhaps you have awaited the results of a job interview or served as a member of a volunteer fire department or the power company's emergency preparedness team awaiting some catastrophe that wipes out a region's electricity. Maybe you've watched the clock while wondering whether your lovestruck teenager would make it home from a date by midnight.

The doctor on call has his own kind of waiting, which produces a strange *je ne sais quoi*. Call it tension, but it's more than that. Being on call does not guarantee that you *will* be called away in the middle of your daughter's first dance recital, or your son's first soccer game, or out of the choir loft on Sunday morning, or even away from your fourteenth wedding anniversary dinner. It means, fundamentally, the *potential* for those things to happen. Even if they don't, they *might*, and that's the problem. What did Roosevelt say? "The only thing we have to fear is fear itself." And the beeper.

"On call" means trapped, cornered, nowhere to run, nowhere to hide! It's not the unmistakable fact that you might be called into the hospital for an emergency. That alone could be easily dealt with emotionally. It's not even the certainty that you are responsible for the very lives of not only your own patients, but your partners' patients as well. That responsibility comes with the territory.

71

No, it's none of these things. It's somehow the fact that the beeper can go off the very next instant! That's the killer. It can scare the hell out of you at anytime! You can be in stage IV sleep—then suddenly yanked into consciousness with no warning whatsoever. You can set your beeper to vibrate so that you don't disturb others in the symphony, or church, or at a lecture. Then... bzzzzzzzz! You look like an idiot when you give an audible start, jump out of your seat for no apparent reason, then apologize to everyone as they readjust to allow you to squeeze by knees, step on toes, and maintain your balance with a quick hand to the shoulder or head of the unsuspecting person sitting one row to the front.

There are other well known (to doctors) phenomena associated with taking call. For instance, if you are just completing an emergency laparoscopic salpingostomy for an ectopic pregnancy at 3:00 a.m., after sixty-eight hours of a seventy-two-hour weekend call, your beeper will begin its annoying, plaintive cry as you are removing your scrub gown. You were just wondering if you'd get to go home for three to four hours before the new day starts. The page will concern a hysterical young woman in horrible pain, bleeding heavily, on her way to the ER. She will be named Hysung Ping and will not speak a word of English. In short, you needn't have worried about going home.

However, frenetic activity is not the callee's worst fate. Almost every physician I know would rather stay continuously busy while on call than simply sit waiting for the other shoe to drop. Physicians go through residencies at which they may spend literally years on call every other night. That means you work for about thirty-six hours straight, take maybe twelve off if you're lucky, and then do your thirty-six hours again! You mathematical wizards out there might have figured that comes to roughly 132 hours a week. I bet you didn't realize there were that many hours in the week. Kinda makes forty hours look a bit anemic, doesn't it?

But we can all tell you that as long as you're working every minute, you can get away with it. Sure, you might fall asleep at every red light on the way home, but the old adrenaline's pumpin' if you're taking a bullet out of somebody's pregnant uterus!

No, the problem in residency came when you had thirty minutes of down time at 4:00 a.m. You would fall asleep on the elevator, somnambulate to the call room, and collapse in a heap on the bunk. Revving the engines again when that hideous beeper went off required Herculean strength, self-discipline, and dedication.

In private practice you may not be comatose despite seventy hours on call because you may have slept for several hours at a stretch throughout the weekend. But you dare not try to go home, or to your child's soccer game, or to the circus that night, or to that movie you really wanted to see (the last one having been *Lawrence of Arabia*), because of the dreaded hip attachment. If you're swamped, you never have a chance to give it a thought. If you're not terribly busy, it's torture!

I should also mention some other well-known "call" phenomena. I don't care what the American College of Obstetrics and Gynecology study showed, all of us OBs know that the moon's gravitational force ruptures membranes. Why is this so hard to believe? After all, the moon tosses around multiple quadrillion tons of ocean water without perceptible effort twice each day. Surely a few liters of amniotic fluid should pose little challenge for the lunar forces.

And what about the "hex"? You have not left the hospital building for fifty-six hours. You have just completed a particularly nerve-wracking midforceps delivery, and it was absolutely the last thing you had to do. Then someone asks you if you have anyone else on the way in. Well, forget it, you are hosed! Sometimes, if you pretend not to have heard the question, and you're convincing, the obstetric gods will consider a reprieve. This, however, is extremely rare. Usually, your beeper senses the question and initiates its incessant buzzing or beeping instantaneously. Occasionally, even your spouse, in his/her ardent desire to have you come home, will err and innocently ask the fatal question. *C'est la vie!*

It doesn't matter if you have a conference to attend in the Virgin Islands or you're on the vacation you've waited eight years to enjoy and planned six months in advance. Some emergency with someone, somewhere, will alter the schedule such that you draw the black bean. You just have to take call right then.

Now, you say, that has to work both ways. There must be times that a doctor needs to get off and others alter their schedules to make it possible. Well, that must be the case, but I'll be damned if any of us can ever remember the last time that happened!

I can hear the objections. "Oh, quit griping! You picked this for a living, didn't you?" Well, not exactly. When you apply to medical school, the counselors skip over the part about no sleep, the ugly spectre of too many attorneys without enough to eat, the physical attachment to the obnoxious little box on your hip, the unimaginably political bureaucracies called "hospitals," and the fact that your children ask for identification before they'll open the front door for you.

But they say it builds character. I suppose in a way it does. It certainly drives home the meaning of the word "responsibility" in one context. Some of us, however, took marriage vows that antedated our taking of the Hippocratic oath. While responsibility may well be learned along the path to becoming a reputable physician, it must also be applied to the role of husband and father. The balance is often extremely precarious. The high divorce rate among physicians is often quoted as evidence of their misplaced loyalties, but usually not as evidence of the total lack thereof. Their loyalties just end up right where they were placed on the first day of medical school, with the patient first, last, and foremost.

I firmly believe that the most effective physician is one who has a secure and rewarding family life. His family benefits from his presence almost as much as he benefits from their support. Fostering this environment takes time and learning as well. It took me over six years as a physician to finally understand that when my home number comes up on the digital beeper, I need to make the call the top priority, not the lowest.

So "call" is not a nice word. We learn to deal with it as a fact of life, but we never really like it. All of us know deep inside our beings that radio pagers are instruments of the devil! But in spite of call, and perhaps partially because of call, we learn that responsibility lies at the heart of a successful life.

WORST-CASE SCENARIO

WE'VE ALLUDED BEFORE to the fallible nature of physicians. We need to realize that errors with sweeping consequences can come in many forms. But a strong physician-patient relationship can ameliorate the effects of such errors. In fact, as will be mentioned in "Danger," it is the strength of such a relationship that can avert many of these errors and the lack of such a relationship that may allow things to fall through the cracks.

It was an even busier morning than usual. The bright April sunshine streamed in through the exam room windows. Moving splotches of gold danced over the counters, cabinets, and exam tables. Outside it was cool, breezy, a gorgeous day. All of my patients probably wished they were someplace else, but it was unusual for me to wish I was too.

As I exited the exam room and prepared to dictate my visit notes, I was thinking about the fact that my weekend off and this phenomenal weather might actually coincide, defying known physical laws of obstetrics. Then I caught a glimpse of my nurse putting one of those sticky notes where I couldn't possibly miss it. That almost always meant trouble. My good mood vaporized.

The note simply said, "Call Sarah, urgent," with a phone number. Usually that kind of note would be annoying—which Sarah? What was the problem? Where was her chart? But it wasn't annoyance I felt this time. And I knew perfectly well which Sarah. What could possibly be "urgent," to a person in her almost unimaginable position?

Sarah was a thirty-eight-year-old clinical psychologist married to a corporate attorney. Married for over fifteen years, they were happy, but infertile. Over the course of the last several years they had endured the entire gamut of infertility tests and procedures. Now they had become the living embodiment of the term "advanced reproductive technology," and they were ecstatic over the discovery of their twin pregnancy.

While Sarah was technically of "advanced maternal age" and thus at some increased risk for various complications, in general she was the optimum candidate for pregnancy at this time of life. Strong, healthy, and trim, Sarah balanced her busy work schedule by swimming up to 3,000 meters a day, a near-perfect exercise for pregnancy, even for women with multiple gestations.

Educated about her primary risks of preterm labor and preeclampsia or toxemia, Sarah was totally in tune with her body. She recognized her own uterine contractions, even the subtle ones barely detected on the monitor. She combined her exercise with an optimum diet, and her blood pressure had remained low-normal throughout the pregnancy. Her pelvic ultrasound at eighteen weeks had shown two girls, both growing at the same rate and without abnormality. In short, she had done "swimmingly" through her first twenty-six weeks of gestation.

She had called around midnight at the start of her twenty-seventh week complaining of excruciating left flank pain. When I met her about one in the morning at labor and delivery, I knew there was something serious going on. Her husband was standing on the far side of the bed holding Sarah in his arms. She was twisted toward him and half-sitting, the lower half of her body on the bed.

She was still for just that one moment when I walked in, her teeth clenched, face a mask of agony, arms wrapped around her husband's neck. Immediately thereafter she resumed her writhing, pushing away from her husband and falling full onto the bed. She rolled back and forth, pleading, screaming for relief through tears of pain.

Anyone who has ever passed a kidney stone or taken care of anyone who did, recognizes the typical presentation. Almost any other kind of intra-abdominal emergency, from a ruptured appendix to a ruptured cyst or ectopic pregnancy, will cause the patient to curl up on her side and lie as still as possible. With a kidney stone, the patient usually does a good imitation of a largemouth bass flopping around on the dock. (One diagnostic test for abdominal pain is to "accidentally" jostle the gurney on which the patient lies and observe the reaction. The kidney stone patient won't notice, but the intra-abdominal catastrophe patient will scream bloody murder.)

But I knew Sarah. I knew her tears were not all pain, but frustration as well. If there was one thing she didn't like, it was losing control. As a clinical psychologist, she dealt with patients whose problems ran the gamut of the mundane young-mother neuroses to the dangerous borderline personalities. Most of the time, Sarah couldn't afford to do anything other than run steady and true on an even keel. To be this out of control was painful physically and emotionally.

After some reassurance about the safety of narcotic pain relievers at twenty-six weeks of pregnancy and the importance of avoiding a seriously preterm twin delivery at almost any cost, Sarah agreed to IV morphine. Her pelvic exam was not too worrisome with respect to cervical change, and despite her agonized thrashing about, delivery did not look to be an immediate concern. We made plans for the usual kidney ultrasound and one shot IVP (intravenous pyelogram), which I felt would surely reveal her kidney stone.

Her pain improved markedly after the morphine. Her urine showed no blood whatsoever. By two hours after arrival, she had no pain at all. While this was somewhat atypical of a stone, we agreed to not pursue any further testing unless there was a recurrent episode. We gave her the usual instruction about how to strain her urine, since she had probably passed the stone into her bladder when the pain stopped, and sent her home with some prophylactic antibiotics.

I saw Sarah the following week, and except for a dull, intermittent ache in the flank, she was doing fine. The twins continued to grow concordantly (at the same rate), and we discussed her cutting back at the office. We also took the necessary steps to set up twice-per-day home uterine-contraction monitoring via a device with which Sarah could transfer her monitoring strips over the phone. The subsequent record could be faxed to us as needed, or more usually, a computer graphic was produced weekly to indicate any patterns of increasingly frequent contractions.

It was only three days later when I saw her again. Unfortunately, to my consternation, it was in a fourth-floor room on the high-risk OB wing. Her hair was disheveled and soaked from perspiration. She was more pale than usual, if that's possible for a redhead. The effect of the narcotics had given her hazel eyes a glazed appearance in the dimly lit room. Her small swimmer's frame, despite the broad shoulders, looked overwhelmed by the size of her protruberant belly. Her husband, Harold, was sitting on the other side of the bed, holding her left hand in both of his. He was balding, medium build, glasses, worried. Maybe a little angry, but not overtly so.

My associate had admitted her this time. She'd come in around 3:00 a.m. with the same violently intense flank pain. Sarah had continued to swim long distances each day, and I had agreed. But the pain seemed totally unrelated to physical activity. It awakened her from a sound sleep and came on like a freight train, easing for a while but then returning in relentless waves. My partner had already set her up for the ultrasound and the X-ray, and they were coming to get her soon.

The pain once again was on the way to resolution, much as it had been ten days previously. But as agreed, I felt it important to get to the bottom of this now. Again, her urine was negative for blood or infection. Her white blood count was normal. She had no fever. Her symptoms could go along with pyelonephritis, or kidney infection; however, her lab work was incompatible. A kidney stone still seemed the most likely etiology of her pain.

While we talked and Harold took what was to become a long list of notes on a legal pad, the X-ray tech arrived with the gurney to take her down into the bowels of the hospital, through the tunnel across the parking lot, and then up into the main building where most of the imaging equipment was located. I rode the elevator down with them and gave her a quick hug when we reached my floor, promising to come discuss the results with her as soon as I had them.

It was several hours later when I walked into their room. She was in bed, but fully dressed and holding a 4x4 gauze over the site where her IV had just been removed. Pain obviously gone, she gave her trademark big smile.

"So, am I outta here? Did they see the stone?"

Her face changed slowly as she looked at mine. Harold took his feet down off the bed and muted the TV with the remote. Without comment, he picked up his legal pad off the window ledge.

"It doesn't look like a stone, Sarah. There appears to be a growth of some sort on your left kidney. This one looks like it might be fairly large since it distorts the image of the ureter, but we'll need a CAT scan or MRI to get a better look." Now Sarah and Harold are well-read, intelligent people, and my use of the term "growth" was pretty transparent to them.

"Are you telling me that I have a kidney tumor?"

"You certainly might, or at least the two studies you had today were suggestive of that. But even if it's true, malignant tumors of the kidney in your age group are almost unheard of. Our problem is going to be keeping your babies on the inside until they're ready to breathe on their own."

Sarah was reaching for a Kleenex, the first shiny tears trickling from the corners of her eyes. Harold spoke for the first time.

"How do you *know* for a fact that it's not malignant?" he said, pen poised over his legal pad.

"First, we need a urology consult, and I imagine he'll want a tissue diagnosis. By that I would mean a needle biopsy normally, but we really should talk to Urology first and follow up on the results of the CAT scan I have scheduled tomorrow."

"But isn't a biopsy dangerous? I mean what about bleeding? What about the twins? Could there be something wrong with them too? Could this deal be hereditary? What if it *is cancer*? If it is I want it *out* right now! No waiting for... " He was getting more and more excited as each new possibility occurred to him.

"Hold on there a minute!" I interrupted. "We don't know she has a tumor. If she does, it is in all probability benign and won't affect anything except possibly to further increase her risk of preterm labor. If that is the case, and she goes into preterm labor, we have medicines to deal with that."

I sat on the end of her bed and grabbed a tennis-shoed foot.

"I want you to stay off of these for awhile. We can do the CAT scan as an outpatient, and then you can see my buddy the urologist the following day. It was about time for you to quit work in any event." I gave her foot a good-natured dog shake. "Look, it's gonna be all right. If something bad were to happen it could hurt my reputation, and I'll not have that!" That got a little smile out of her. Her husband did not look terribly reassured.

I don't believe she even got the CAT scan as an outpatient. The pain returned the next night, and she was right back on the high-risk antepartum unit. I do remember that the CAT scan did not look like the usual fatty benign renal tumor. In fact, the radiologist told me it looked quite a bit like the BAD DISEASE. The urologist and I agreed that an MRI would be even more helpful.

The evening after the MRI, I spent nearly two hours in Sarah's room. Harold was calm, and his questions were logical and well thought out. Sarah was unusually quiet, and although her questions were less frequent, they always centered around the twins. It rapidly became clear that slightly different priorities were emerging.

Harold cut to the chase.

"So, there definitely is a large tumor in the left kidney, and it doesn't look like the kind of benign tumor that would be more common in her age group?"

"That is true," I said simply.

"Okay, let's take the worst-case scenario. Let's just assume this is cancer. What do we do?" Sarah was crying quietly again. The lights in the room were off, and the sky was in that final gray stage before true darkness, a good hour after sunset. The parking lot lights were stark;

they silhouetted Harold in his position on the windowsill, his legal pad over one crossed leg.

"We'll have to talk more with Brian (the urologist), but I do know this kidney will have to be removed. It is extremely unlikely that this tumor could be removed and also save any normal kidney. There is now little function in the involved kidney, and the surgery to remove the entire kidney would be safer, quicker, and with less blood loss than trying just to remove the tumor. Whether or not the tumor is... "

"When?" Sarah said. Just "when?"

There was one of those awkward silences. All I could tell them for sure was that surgery was likely to precipitate preterm labor. Twins at twenty-eight weeks do better now than ever before in NICUs (neonatal intensive care units), but they also die 10–20 percent of the time and are permanently damaged in some way a greater percentage of time than that. I recommended that we wait at least another month, until thirty-two weeks, if possible. That would give the twins an excellent chance of undamaged survival even if Sarah went into preterm labor.

"Why not wait until the twins are really ready and do both surgeries at the same time? Wouldn't that be best for the twins?" Sarah wanted to know. Almost without pause, Harold asked if it wouldn't be better for Sarah to get it out as soon as possible. Like tomorrow, for instance.

How's this for a potential no-win situation? Do a nephrectomy ASAP and possibly lose twins who were ten years in the making. Given the couple's infertility, that might close the book on their chance to reproduce. Or, delay the surgery, deal with the preterm labor, which was already worsening, in the hope of getting healthy twins, but possibly leave the patient's malignancy to spread over the next four to six weeks.

I left the room with a clear message from the patient. Do what must be done to give the twins the best chance. I left the room with a clear message from the patient's husband. Do what must be done to save my wife's life.

After further discussion with the urologist and his partners, we decided that the odds were still way in favor of this being a benign tumor. Consequently, I would do what was necessary to avoid delivery until thirty-four weeks. We would then perform a cesarean section, the twins would have an excellent chance, and we would delay removal of the kidney until six weeks postpartum when Sarah's blood volume had recovered.

Harold was difficult to convince. Our argument was that if malignant, despite the lack of distant metastases, a tumor this size would surely have already ruptured the renal capsule and delay in removal would do little to prolong the inevitable. Harold wasn't buying it.

As it turned out, after discharge, Harold and Sarah got a second opinion at the medical school. The chief of urology there felt that there was a significant chance of malignancy with this tumor's appearance and he recommended immediate removal.

We resolved the controversy the only way we could, the way all men do in the long run; we did what we were told. Harold by his wife, me by my patient. We agreed to delay the surgery until at least thirty-two weeks, give the twins a good chance at normalcy if we were forced to deliver them, but in the hope of keeping them in afterwards for at least another month.

Sarah continued to swim over the next several weeks despite increasing discomfort. She continued to be the model patient, and her uterine contractions, while increasingly frequent, were not enough to prove dangerous.

I don't think I'll ever forget the image of a small-framed, naked woman with a huge abdomen lying halfway on her back and halfway on her side, chest arched unnaturally over a roll. Her arms were extended over her head, endotracheal tube taped into her mouth, eyes taped closed. Fetal heart tones were fine as we prepped and draped her flank.

The surgery to remove the kidney went well. The pathology did not. There is no easy way to deliver the news that someone has what everyone prayed they did not. There is no easy way to tell a loving, devoted husband that his mate has an incurable cancer. It is a death knell. It is the end of the world as he knows it. It is a betrayal, in a way. It is incomprehensible. We told Harold we would have to await the final pathology, but the frozen section looked very worrisome. We told him that the surgery had gone as well as could be expected. He was tearful and silent.

Sarah went to the antepartum ICU. She was on a special subcutaneous terbutaline pump to keep her contractions under control. There was an epidural in place to help with post-op pain. As it turned out, it was too low to be very helpful, and her next few days were miserable. She was in and out of a narcotic stupor, battling with IVs, bladder catheter, nausea, itching, and almost unimaginable discomfort at thirty-two weeks with twins and a foot long, muscle-splitting flank incision.

Then came a chain of snafus. Three days after the operation, a well-meaning floor nurse called the psych-social worker because Sarah had been difficult and demanding since surgery. The floor nurse neglected to ask either me or the urologist if this was okay; in fact, neither of us had yet been informed of the final path report, which had just come back. The social worker read the report, then interrupted Sarah's visit with a friend, asked the visitor to leave, and questioned Sarah as to how she might help her deal with her anger.

Anger about what? Sarah asked.

Why, your anger about your cancer, of course!

I got there about ten minutes later, having told my nurse to cancel the remaining two hours of the afternoon. Sarah was inconsolable. In a cowardly sort of fashion it was now much easier for me. I sat on the bed and held Sarah in my arms as she rocked back and forth like a small child. She reminded me of my own little girl when I try to quiet the wracking sobs that accompany a particularly frightening nightmare.

In the ensuing days I spent many more hours with Sarah and Harold. While Urology would give them the straight facts, I would come by to reinterpret them in a better light. When they told her it was a particularly rare form of renal sarcoma, I would tell her at least it hadn't broken through the renal capsule. When they told her it could already have spread elsewhere through her blood stream, I told her there was no evidence that it had, and as far as anyone but God knew, she might well already be cured.

We delayed discussion of further therapy until after her delivery. She did well once off the preterm labor medicines, and just as soon as she had almost fully recovered from her flank incision, it was time for her cesarean section. We got all the way to thirty-six weeks, and twin girls were born without a hitch.

How can one describe the melancholy surrounding the joyful delivery of long-awaited twins to a loving mother who has been told there is a less than 5 percent chance that she will witness their second birthday? In the weeks that followed, Sarah began a journal and video tapes of instructions for the girls to be played as they reached anticipated birthdays and expected goals all the way to adulthood. She tried to think of herself as cured and take one day at a time, but it was difficult in light of the facts she faced. The local chemotherapy doctors told her there was no effective regimen for her disease and recommended no treatment unless metastases showed up. Sarah and Harold both wanted the most aggressive treatment available. I agreed they should go to M.D. Anderson in Houston for a second opinion.

When I saw the Post-it note, I just couldn't imagine what was urgent. Surely she had not already developed a distant symptom, and it was too far out from her c-section to be a complication. We had spoken only two days ago on her return from Houston. They had agreed that the only treatment would be toxic, experimental, unlikely to have any benefit, and would adversely affect large blocks of her few remaining healthy months. What could possibly be urgent?

I dialed the phone and braced myself.

"Hi, gorgeous! What's so urgent." I tried to be my usual jovial self.

"I'm not gonna die. How's that for urgent!!" You could just see her beaming without a video phone.

"Excuse me?" I couldn't hide my bewilderment.

"You were right to begin with. You told me it wasn't

gonna be cancer before the surgery. Then you told me to think 'cured' afterwards." She was giddy.

"I'm still lost, Sarah."

"M.D. Anderson just called. They reviewed the slides. I don't have cancer. They've all reviewed them down there and nobody thinks it's malignant!!"

"That's fantastic!" I screamed, drawing inquiring looks from my patient checking out, the receptionist, and the nurse.

"Apparently it's a rare type of tumor that looked confusing under the microscope. So can you believe it?"

"I believe it, Sarah. Go swim some laps. I've got new energy for work!"

The sun was still streaming in the windows. It really was springtime after all. Once more I had learned that *nothing* is written in stone, it's okay to count my chicks before they hatch, it's not over till the fat lady sings, the rain in Spain falls mainly on the plain, whiskers on kittens and blue satin sashes are among my favorite things, and it really does help to whistle a happy tune whenever you feel afraid.

SAMANTHA

BEING A PHYSICIAN is not just another job. It's a commitment to doing the utmost to maintain and restore the health of our patients—the health that is not merely physical or emotional, but the interweaving of both that makes people what they are when they're at their best.

The following is a very personal experience. I feel that I can relate it now only because it happened so long ago, but also because I feel so strongly that the essence of the physician-patient relationship is in grave danger in this country today. I don't expect that the depth of feeling I recall here could—or should—be brought to a doctor's every relationship with a patient. But I do know that in this patient's ordeal, I learned about loss. I learned about compassion. I learned about love in a real sense. And I learned that averting suffering is a worthy goal in life.

She was twenty-six, maybe twenty-seven years old. She didn't look it, of course, lying there soaked in sweat. Her hospital gown clung to her rail-thin frame as though only fossilized remains were concealed. Her once-porcelain skin was bruised horribly, every inch of her neck and forearms covered with splotches of purple, green, and yellow. Her most recent IV site was, I think she knew, to be her final one. The bulky bandage on her left upper chest protruded awkwardly from the neck of the faded blue gown. The subclavian IV tubing lay as limp as her spirit across the pillow. No, she didn't look twenty-six. But it wasn't that she looked older, either. She just didn't look right. She just didn't look right at all.

Her long brown hair had long since been lost. Only those of us who had seen her in years past could even visualize the beautiful girl she had been. The chemotherapy had seemed to go on forever. Methotrexate, cytoxan, adriamycin (the Red Death, we called it): she'd had it all, in multiple courses. This last time in, though, was the worst. Maybe it was the worst because of the bleed into her head with the resulting loss of movement on the left side, or maybe because of the radiation to her already denuded scalp, but surely because she and all the rest of us knew she wouldn't be leaving again.

It had happened like most cases of fatal choriocarcinoma. A happy, bright, optimistic woman of twenty-three had become pregnant a little before she had planned. She and her boyfriend had decided to keep the baby and commit their lives to each other, but as fate would have it, the young lady began spotting and cramping at about seven weeks' gestation and subsequently lost the pregnancy.

Because she was so early on when the spotting began, the doctor had told her that bedrest was her only option. Despite compliance, her cramping and bleeding had rapidly worsened one night about three in the morning. The girl was frightened and just ready to head for the emergency room when the cramping stopped abruptly and the bleeding trailed off to only spotting again. She called the doctor, who told her that she had probably passed all the tissue and completed her miscarriage. Had she saved the tissue? Well, no. No one had told her that was important. He reassured her that it was okay, but he needed to see her back in the office in three to four weeks.

Her boyfriend could hardly hide his relief at the turn of events. She, on the other hand, was devastated. How could the loss of the life they had made together mean so little to him?

He said that wasn't it. She wasn't being fair and he was just being realistic. She told him to get out. He did.

The loss of her pregnancy, as well as her dream of the handsome prince, was almost too much to bear. Her depression lasted for several months, but with the love and support of her parents and her friends, she began to recover. Her parents owned a successful winery in Sonoma and consequently were quite well off. They sent her and a girlfriend on a six-week tour of Europe, where they used their Eurail passes to extinction. They did Portugal, Spain,

France, Italy, and then left the coast to take in Switzerland, Austria, Germany, Holland, Denmark, and then back to London. Her only regret was not getting to see the Greek Isles. But there was always time for that, right?

The appointment. That follow-up appointment. She'd forgotten all about that. Now it had been over a year. She really should go back to see him, and her periods hadn't really been all that regular, had they? In fact, she couldn't really remember when the last one had occurred. Wasn't it back in the summer, before she'd left for Europe? Oh well, she'd just make an appointment now and get in to see him.

The doctor had been pleasant enough. Hadn't she gotten the letters he'd sent her about follow-up? No? Well, we'll just set things right today. Did she have a current sexual partner? No? Not since the miscarriage? She didn't really know when her last period was?

His exam had been routine. He told her that he felt nothing abnormal. But would she please leave a urine specimen in the bathroom off the exam room?

She was writing her check at the front desk when the doctor came up beside her and gently placed his left hand on her forearm. Could she step into the office just for a second? He had something they needed to discuss.

She told me that she often thought of that afternoon. She had sat across the desk from him. The guest chair had faced west, but she could gaze out the picture windows to the north and catch a magnificent view of the bay. The sunlight was streaming over the whitecaps bouncing off the straight white walls of Alcatraz and bathing the vast expanse of green between the marina and the yacht club in a golden afternoon glow. The whole window framed an idyllic scene, which she remembered as a rainbow palette of color given life by the wind, with soaring gulls, billowing sails, and ocean spray on the breakwaters.

He was telling her that her pregnancy test was positive. She told me that she clearly remembered giggling inside, anticipating his retraction when he learned of her celibacy since the miscarriage. Then as she glanced out the window again, she remembered that he already had asked about that. She started to get a little scared with the realization that the test wasn't in error.

After the word "cancer," she pretty much tuned out everything. She hadn't meant to, but she'd suddenly remembered the Greek Isles, and the look on her boyfriend's face the first time they had made love, and the fact that she hadn't sent either of her parents cards for Mother's or Father's Day this year. These things she told to me.

Eventually she was to fully understand what gestational trophoblastic disease entailed. There were no blood pregnancy assays for human chorionic gonadotropin (HCG) back then. The urine tests were also markedly less sensitive. Today a positive pregnancy test will pick up only 25mIU of HCG in the urine, and this only ten days after conception. Back then, the urine tests were sensitive to about 10,000 mIU of HCG, or 400-fold less sensitive. They would pick up a normal pregnancy no earlier than six weeks from the last period or about thirty days after conception. Unfortunately for the patient, this meant that the presence of a GTN (gestational trophoblastic neoplasm) could not be detected until it was advanced enough to produce relatively high levels of HCG, its marker hormone.

GTN is a particularly tragic trick of fate. It develops only after a spontaneous miscarriage, a genetically abnormal pregnancy called a "mole," or after term pregnancy. The placenta is normally an invasive organ. No one yet understands why it normally halts its invasion of the human female when partially burrowed in the wall of the uterus.

As one in fifty Asian women and one in one thousand Caucasian women know, however, it doesn't always stop.

The chorion, or outer layer of the placental tissue, may become abnormally aggressive, grow through the wall of the uterus, and/or spread its malignant cells to distant parts of the body such as lung, liver, and brain. Prior to the 1960s, this disease was uniformly and rapidly fatal. By 1975 it was almost completely curable, if detected early. *If* detected early.

Today patients with this disease might be handled

largely as outpatients, but at that time it was routine to admit them for a full work-up. She arrived in old bell-bottom jeans and a peasant blouse, carrying a floral carpet bag containing the worldly possessions she thought essential for such a venture. I had seen her walk by the nurses' station from the elevator, accompanied by a statuesque middle-aged woman in a stunning red dress who wore jewelry in a way that said she was quite accustomed to such luxuries.

It was that first day that I was assigned to her care as a second-year resident. We were at the university hospital up on the hill overlooking Kezar Stadium and Golden Gate Park beyond. She'd had her blood drawn already and had just returned from X-ray when I stepped in. She was an impossibly beautiful girl, or maybe I've just made her that way in my memory. She sat on the edge of the bed clutching a large, once-white, shabby teddy bear to her chest.

She looked up as I entered the room, flipping her long chestnut hair over her shoulder with just a toss of her head. (They must teach beautiful girls how to do that just right, somewhere.) Her hazel eyes seemed to sparkle, perhaps a little moist, as they caught the late afternoon sun through the window. She was now attired in the infamous faded blue hospital gown, open to the rear, but had managed to hang on to her tight bell bottoms.

I introduced myself to her and her mother and asked if this was a good time to talk to her for a few minutes. Her mother commented that I looked awfully young. The patient, almost whispering, said that anytime was a good time now, wasn't it? The mother reached out and put her hand on her daughter's arm. "Stop that, honey. It's gonna work out, you'll see." Her glance said she wasn't that sure of her words, or of me.

The rest of that interview was pretty much like any other at which a parent is present, i. e., the mother constantly answered questions directed at her daughter, continuing her lifelong role as protector. It was impossible to inject any levity into the situation. But despite the patient's intermittent crying, she and I shared a private smile at the expense of her mother when the lady turned

91

her attention to rooting through her oversized purse for some vaccination records.

As any doctor might have expected, the chest X-ray showed multiple "cannon ball" metastases throughout the lung fields. Her urine collection showed levels well over the 100,000 mark needed to assign her to the poor prognosis group. By the time the next day's CAT scan results were available, it was no surprise to anyone that her liver was a mine field as well. Only the brain scan was normal.

Despite this troubling picture, we were able to give the patient some hope. People do respond remarkably well to modern chemotherapy with this disease. In that no gross tumor could be imaged in the uterus and a D&C was unrevealing, surgery was not proposed as part of her treatment. In fact, the appearance of her metastases was so classic that biopsy data was not even felt necessary before starting treatment.

I was on the oncology service for three months, so I managed to see her over several hospitalizations. She'd be in for four to six days, home for a week or two, and back again for treatment.

We residents mixed the Red Death ourselves so as to absolve the nurses of any responsibility should there be a dosing error. We mixed it under a venti-hood with masks and gloves on so that not even fumes of the potent agent could reach our tissues. It always struck me as bizarre to take all these precautions against any possible accidental exposure and then march into this young woman's room, hook up her IV, and pump this toxin into her with a smile on my face.

She took it quite well. After her initial terror, she would joke with me about how little she feared chemo, having been forced to drink the family's wine for nearly three decades! But the vomiting was God-awful, and the phenothiazine derivatives never really helped unless we gave her enough to knock her out for a few hours. Often I would be rushing to finish one of the hundreds of tasks required daily to evaluate and treat the thirty to forty cancer patients on the floor at any one time, when I would peek in her door and find her sleeping on her side with her arms around that ragged bear. I remember feeling guilty that I found myself praying for her recovery and not for any of the other patients in my charge, most of whom were twenty to forty years her senior.

It took only one admission for me to look forward to her next. She responded better than we could have hoped, her HCG dropping quickly and dramatically after the first few treatments. Her chest X-ray cleared, her liver enzymes returned to normal, and those of us new and naive began to feel proud of ourselves for defeating this scourge.

She looked just as gorgeous without any hair to me. She used to love to return to the floor unscheduled, wearing a new wig and sunglasses, and fool the nurses who knew her so well into believing she was whoever she claimed to be that day.

I never saw her tearful again after that first day. Never. Even after the third and fourth relapses over two years later, she maintained her ebullient determination. Always her HCG titers would drop, but never back to the normal range, and each time the descent was slower. We used to present her graphs in conference as examples of the relentless nature of the disease.

While the chemotherapy took only a few days, her weakened immune system always permitted some viral or bacterial invader to take up residence briefly before being evicted by antibiotics. Thus, her hospital stays toward the spring of 1984 became longer; the next-to-last time she came, she was hospitalized for two weeks.

Her friends stopped visiting toward the end. I don't know whether their lives had forced them to move on or they just couldn't stand to watch death's inexorable approach. Incredibly, I found myself frequently stopping to sit with her at the end of a gruesome day to cheer myself up. Sometimes we'd sit for forty-five minutes and talk of our respective plans. She'd always ask after my wife. When I'd drag myself into her room after seventy-two hours awake, she'd reassure me that one day it would all be worth it. She'd talk of her plans for the Greek Isles, finally deciding that living there would be better than just visiting. So she worked out an elaborate schedule for the next summer that would end with her finding some Greek god and trampling grapes naked on a hillside in the sun.

When I left her room that Friday after the stroke, I couldn't stop crying. I'd controlled myself in the room and even laughed when she summoned her miniscule strength to imitate the creature from the black lagoon, drawing attention to the drooping left side of her once pretty face. We'd held hands most of that last visit. Her family was nowhere to be seen, but it's possible that I had simply missed their visits.

I told her I still wanted to see her winery before she headed for Greece next summer. She promised me a tour and attempted a smile. I don't know if either of us really knew we'd never see the other again, but I kissed her forehead as I snuggled her bear up against her. She closed her eyes and said she needed a nap.

I was off that weekend. I remember we went up to Stinson Beach and basked in the sun and the sea air. In retrospect, I'm not sure I even thought of her much that Saturday at the beach. I was too busy soaking up life for myself.

Monday she was gone. I went by her room in the morning around seven expecting to see that old bear and his lifelong charge and instead found an emaciated elderly Chinese woman with terminal ovarian cancer. At first I thought perhaps she'd been moved to the ICU for life support. But then I realized she would never have permitted that.

When I got home that night about nine, there was a case of wine on the coffee table. My wife wondered who it was from. The tag said simply that this was "just in case we didn't get a chance to take that tour." I sank to the couch and, in a quite unmanly fashion, burst into tears. My wife pulled my head to her lap as I fell over and surrendered to the sobs.

I guess, maybe, I was a little bit in love with her.

Her name was Samantha.

MUM'S THE WORD

WHILE PHYSICIANS DEAL with both the technical and the emotional aspects of their patients' care, they must also deal with constraints placed on them by the very structure of that physician-patient relationship. Preserving confidentiality is of course paramount to a trusting relationship, but much as it can with attorney-client privilege, that confidentiality can lead one into ethical dilemmas.

Many of these dilemmas might seem more easily resolved by breaching the confidence in order to prevent further injury, but the doctor must choose, almost without fail, to err in favor of the sacred trust he has established with his charge via the Hippocratic Oath.

My mistake was in agreeing to see the patient in the first place. Seeing your wife's best friend professionally is almost, but not quite, as stupid as seeing your wife professionally. While it may be unwise a priori, it is particularly unwise in a situation such as this one.

After all, my first helpful little bit of medical advice for Sharon had come several years before when her little boy, then four, had flown off of their new swing set like an unguided missile. My wife and I had the misfortune of being there in the back yard at the time.

Being the swell guy that I am, I cursorily examined the screaming child and assured her mother that neither of her son's injured arms were fractured. Apparently my gynecologic training had obliterated any memories of the green-stick fractures common in toddlers who fall onto their outstretched arms. Needless to say, after a sleepless night of whimpering, a set of X-rays, and an exam by a qualified pediatric orthopedic surgeon, Kevin got to wear casts on both arms for the next six weeks.

While our relationship remained cordial, the red flags should have gone up when my wife discovered that her

95

friend's recent insurance switch did not allow her to see the OB/GYN she had seen for years and suggested that she see me instead. Kevin was five by then, and our friends were anxious to multiply but had evidently been having difficulty with the "be fruitful" part. Well, again like the swell guy that I am, I offered to see Sharon for insurance only, fully realizing that this probably meant "free" where infertility was concerned.

In the course of the first visit, Sharon's history revealed Kevin to be a miracle baby, in that her husband's semen analysis proved him to be sterile. There must have been some reason for the evaporation of his sperm-making capabilities, but none was offered.

Right there, had this not been my wife's best friend, I would have questioned her story. But no, I blindly accepted this history as the gospel. A discussion of donor insemination ensued, and shortly thereafter arrangements were made for frozen donor insemination from a reputable national bank. The sperm from the donor whose description Sharon and her husband had chosen was flown into town in liquid nitrogen, thawed, and placed high in the uterus via a transcervical catheter on the appropriate day before, and again after, the day of ovulation. This was done since the sperm can live in the female genital tract for forty-eight to seventy-two hours, while the egg only survives for up to twenty-four hours. Ovulation was controlled by injection of the hormone that signals egg release after confirming its readiness with vaginal ultrasound.

Again, the first cycle should have been a warning of bad karma. Naturally the appropriate day had fallen on a weekend so that I, rather than the nurse, had given the shot. Sharon's injection site became extremely red and swollen, like none other I had ever seen. Well, it was either an allergic reaction to the serum or an abscess. I treated her with oral antibiotics, and I resolved over several painful days while I reassured Sharon as to the infinitesimal possibility of it happening again.

Of course, it did happen again the following cycle, and luckily my embarrassment was lessened by the fact that this cycle she conceived. Everyone was ecstatic! Errors of judgment with respect to green-stick fractures were forgotten by all! Now, like the swell guy I am, I agreed to continue seeing Sharon as an obstetric patient. Her husband had just lost his job. Insurance-only status saved them money, and so of course I agreed to see her, despite feeling vaguely uncomfortable.

Her first OB visit was like thousands of others. Ultrasound revealed a 16mm fetus with a beating heart, and we were all thrilled. We went through the usual first OB visit discussions covering review of medications, diet, exercise, travel, sex, and antenatal testing when appropriate. She had the usual Pap smear, group B strep culture and routine labs. All went well. Everybody was happy and relieved.

Then her HIV test came back positive. *Whoa, what did you just say? Your wife's best friend's HIV test came back positive? Your wife's monogamous, God-fearing, never had a blood transfusion, pure as the driven snow best friend's HIV test came back positive?*

Read major problem here. Read patient confidentiality above all else. Read a terrified young woman who can't explain to her best friend why she seems to be crying all the time. Read doctor who can't tell his wife why her best friend seems to be crying all the time.

You may take several oaths in your life, and if you're lucky, they'll never come in conflict with one another. But try looking the mother of your children in the face and telling her that you have no idea why her best friend is so upset. Does it have anything to do with her pregnancy? *Well, yes, sort of. Well, no, not really. Well, I really can't say. What I mean is, I have no idea!*

You find yourself lying to the one person in the world to whom you swore you would never lie. And yet you also swore that without the patient's permission you would never reveal anything told you in confidence. Even a dense physician can start to understand the wisdom of never treating one's own family and close friends.

Now, I told her first thing that this was probably a false positive. The HIV screen is only that, a screen, and many previous viral infections could have caused cross-reacting antibodies. Besides, with her history, she'd had

97

no possible exposure. We'd simply have to wait the ten days (which happened to be the ten days prior to Christmas) for the confirmatory western blot to return totally negative, as it surely would, and then we could ignore the screen results.

The western blot came back positive for every single antibody tested. In fact it even carried a statement that read, "This patient has been exposed to the HIV virus and should be considered actively infected." It didn't read "might" or "could" have been exposed. It said she *had been exposed.*

"Shocked" is not adequate to describe my feelings. I called the lab and got verbal confirmation of the written result I had already received by fax. Now what was I going to do? How do I tell her this at ten weeks of pregnancy? How do I tell her there's a 25 percent chance her baby will be infected? How do I casually work into the conversation the fact that her husband and six-year-old son may already be infected?

I talked to Sharon and her husband in person at my office. I was as gentle as I know how to be, but it was brutal nevertheless. I'm sure they visualized, as I did, the spectre of a fetus doomed to die and their son without a mother sometime in the near future. When the tears and sobs abated for a moment, a new story came out.

They were sorry that they'd lied to me, but Kevin was not their own child naturally, at least not her husband's. He had always been sterile, and the boy, in fact, had been conceived by artificial insemination as well; except that seven years before, the sperm was fresh, not frozen-donor, and none of the donors were tested for AIDS at that time.

This little bit of information qualified as a bomb shell! While the western blot is considered definitive, I sent both their samples to another lab for independent confirmation. This was only a formality, since I had never heard of a 100 percent positive western blot being in error unless the wrong person's blood was tested. I extracted the appropriate information about which doctors had helped her in the past and learned that two had treated her using the sperm of eight donors in all.

Immediately we began the time-intensive task of

tracking all the donors down by phone. Only one was still in Texas. The other seven lived all over the United States, Canada, and Europe. Unfortunately, before even beginning the search, I knew what the results would be. Without a doubt, my wife's best friend would die young.

Miraculously, after about a week, we had tracked down all but one donor. All were healthy, and all had had negative HIV tests negative within the last year. The final donor was in the USAF assigned to the Aleutians. It took to the last minute of nine days to get the clearance to confirm that he too was healthy and had recently obtained a negative HIV test.

So, was there some more history lurking here? Unfortunately, I had to approach that directly with Sharon, who was of course offended. No, neither she nor her husband were involved with any drugs or deviant sexual practices. Now my wife's best friend was more upset than ever, and the pressure from my wife was becoming unbearable.

The following day, the day after Christmas that particular year, the second laboratory's results on Sharon and her husband came back. Not only was their western blot totally negative, but even their screens were negative! I was flabbergasted. I had brought this woman almost to the brink of suicide, according to both her and her husband's accounts. I had waited for the supposedly foolproof confirmatory test before even discussing the need for further testing of her husband and son. For a little while at least, I had devastated a family.

After being flabbergasted, I was furious. It took almost a week of phone calls to all sorts of people at this national lab before I could get any inkling of an explanation. It turned out that the screening test, although reported as positive or negative, is actually an antibody titer.

If the results are greater than 1.0, it is reported as positive. Period. No borderlines, no repeats, no maybes. Sharon's result had been 1.09. It turns out that most positives that are true findings have numbers like 4.0 to 20.0. This information, however, was not available to me as the clinician because the lab felt all suspicious screens should receive further testing.

I called the patient and relayed the good news about the second lab's results. A third lab later independently confirmed the negative results. Finally, in return for this information, I was freed to let my wife in on the events of the last several months. I can clearly recall the weight lifting from my shoulders.

Questions of confidentiality are a constant in the physician's life, especially given the rather intimate nature of gynecology.

Another time I was seeing a young woman, thirty weeks pregnant, on a routine visit. I commented on the bruises liberally distributed across her upper arms, her throat, her breast, her buttocks.

She started to cry. I asked her directly if her husband did this to her. "Yes," she finally choked out. "He's really gentle, he just flies into a rage when he's drunk and I don't want to make love, or when the baby cries, or when he's having trouble at work. Please don't say anything. He loves me, he really does, but, but... he'd *kill me* if he knew I'd said anything!"

Well, an ordinary problem of confidentiality, you say? Do you report this to the police? Do you call a battered woman's shelter? Can you do any of that when the patient begs you not to?

How about throwing this in the pot? Her husband is the son of a physician with whom I trained for many years and consider to be one of my closest friends. "No," the patient responds when I ask. "My father-in-law knows nothing about this, and he never will!"

I've got an obligation to protect my patient's health. Preventing further battery falls within the scope of that obligation, does it not? Well, not if your intervention is refused, it doesn't.

Oh, I did the usual things. I gave her the information about area shelters. I urged her to dump the "gentle" jerk that day, right then, right that minute! Take your little boy and don't ever go back there! But she went home like most do, convinced that she was trapped. Who knows? She may be lucky. She went on to have the baby and is now pregnant with a third. She tells me he only cuffs her around once every few months now, but then he isn't home much.

The temptation to involve her physician father-in-law is almost overwhelming. I know him to be a decent, caring man, and I would have presumed a good father. Surely he has no idea of what is going on or the potential danger in which his grandchildren could find themselves! But what if he *does* know or suspects? No, breaking a confidentiality in any other situation than direct danger to a minor is always the wrong choice. I kept my mouth shut.

Then there's the thirty-four-year-old North Dallas beauty. Tennis player, Junior League, circle at church, two kids, Chevy Suburban, and now condyloma acuminatum, or "venereal warts."

"What should I do? Could I tell my husband I got this fifteen years ago?"

"Did you?"

"Well, no," she says with a sheepish grin.

"Do you have another sexual partner currently?"

"Well, I know it sounds too trite, but yes, I've been sleeping with the tennis pro at the club. Couldn't you just treat me and then, if it comes up, talk with my husband and tell him it's been dormant for years?"

While this seems a little more heinous than writing a note to the airline documenting the illness for which the patient tells you she missed her flight (despite the fact that she never contacted your office at the time), the principle is the same. Lying about something and keeping something confidential are two different things. I refused the debutante's request, but did tell her our conversation would remain sacrosanct. If her husband should query me, he would be directed to discuss the matter further with his wife.

Yesterday a Middle Eastern patient of mine presented to the office for placement of an IUD. We discussed risks and benefits at length, and realizing that after four children at age thirty she was perhaps an optimum candidate, I agreed to place the IUD.

After the placement, during the vaginal ultrasound to

confirm proper positioning, she mentioned casually that by the way, if her husband knew about this he would slit her throat! (Excuse me, *whose* throat?) Presto change-o, a routine contraceptive visit just became an issue of confidentiality. No billing statements saying "IUD." Questions: Will he be able to feel the string? Will this last until menopause?

An attractive forty-year-old patient desperately wants to be pregnant. She claims to have been unsuccessful at conceiving despite no birth control during her three-year marriage. Her husband, a pilot, never comes with her to any visits or consults. She says it's his schedule. She convinces me that he is unwilling to do the usual screening semen analysis, Besides, why would it be needed? He'd fathered two children in his previous marriage.

Well, why indeed? Her work-up proceeds. She starts on fertility pills to help her ovulate. Despite success with induction of ovulation over the course of several months, she fails to conceive. We perform an HSG, the X-ray to see if the tubes are patent. As often occurs, there is some therapeutic benefit and the patient becomes pregnant the next month. Then the phone call.

"Dr. Thurston?"

"Yes, what can I do for you? And by the way, congratulations!"

"That's what I wanted to talk about. You need to know that I don't want you to mention anything about the infertility at our first obstetric appointment. Is that a problem?"

"Not a problem, but do you mind telling me why not?"

"Well, Harry never wanted to have any more children. He sort of doesn't know about my visits for the last six months."

"Sort of?"

"He thinks I get a lot of yeast infections. So, mum's the word, O.K.?"

I gave her the short course on "Once we practice to deceive, what a tangled web we weave," but I think it was lost on her.

So confidentiality protects the victimized but also the guilty. It solidifies a relationship, which may leave the physician in an uncomfortable position, but ensures that the patient can trust her doctor with things that no one else is allowed to know.

There's an obvious practical benefit to this trust. Once patients learn that they can trust you completely, they will be more likely to reveal factors that lead to accurate diagnosis and treatment. For example, if a patient can tell you that yes, she and her partner practice oral sex, and yes, he sometimes gets fever blisters, then the diagnosis of genital herpes can remain in the "embarrassing" category and not move into the "suspicion of infidelity" category that would result. Catastrophic results can thus be avoided through confidentiality.

Good doctors can be relied upon to be good secret keepers. Even if keeping some secrets is painful or seems ethically wrong at the time, its value to the physician-patient relationship is incalculable.

IT'S A MIRACLE!

PHYSICIANS TEND TO DWELL on their failures more than their successes. I am sure this is related to their Type A, obsessive-compulsive personality profiles. If a patient dies or has serious complications, or even if she just doesn't get what she came to me for in the first place, I can agonize over it for weeks, months, or sometimes years, driving my wife to distraction.

"What about the four-thousand happy, healthy bundles of joy you've helped bring into the world?" she asks. "Think about them now and then!" She is right of course, a given in my marriage. So much is right about this world, from the flowers, to the ocean, to the mountains, to first love, to everlasting love, to the innocence of my five-year-old. We should focus on that from time to time and not dwell on what's wrong in the world.

My job as an obstetrician allows me a very special part in the joy of so many that the anguish of a few should not overshadow it. Recently I had a photograph taken with a woman and her five children, all of whom I delivered. As a part of her family, I can't help but care what happens to her in a very genuine way. There is something intangible but vital in that, something that must not be lost.

A few minutes ago I helped ease out her little head, unwrapped the umbilical cord from around her neck, and then slapped her vigorously on the chest after her mother pushed her the rest of the way into the world. There was no sound for a moment as dad looked through the viewfinder of his video camera, as mom strained to see between her outstretched legs, as the nurse and anesthetist considered their next move, if needed, and as I clamped and cut the cord.

When I swung the baby rapidly from upside down to right side up, she did what almost all babies do to greet the new world—she screamed. Mom started crying quietly and dad yelled, "It's a girl, honey, it's a girl!!" The nurse spread the blanket across the patient's chest, and I gently laid the still wailing, squirming, slippery newborn in her mother's arms.

If you've had a healthy baby, you understand. But unless you're a nurse, midwife, or obstetrician, you've not been able to experience the miracle of new life more than a few times at most. For those of us that have seen it thousands of times, it never loses any of its novelty.

Birth is quite without a doubt the strongest evidence on earth for the existence of God. There are few atheist parents. Those who exist must consciously work to avoid the obvious. It's on their newborn's face as she sleeps. It's on his face when he takes his first steps. It's written all over the smile of accomplishment for simply peeing in the potty! It's there when their kids scream, "It's Daddy!! You're home!!"

My history with Martha went back eight years to a Sunday morning at 3:00 a.m. when I operated on her for a ruptured tubal ectopic pregnancy. Two years later, I delivered her first child—a close call I'll never forget.

Martha had delivered vaginally with no problem. The baby was resting comfortably over in the warmer. But after the delivery of the placenta, she continued to bleed. Her uterus was intermittently boggy, or "atonic," and its failure to contract after a long, hard labor was resulting in her continued hemorrhage. IV Pitocin, IM Methergine, IM prostaglandin f2alpha were all instituted. The joy of having kept her on the planet two years before was slipping from my hands as she bled profusely despite my best efforts. Her terrified husband was escorted from the room as I explained to Martha, who had no epidural, that we would have to put her to sleep to explore the uterus.

After she was out, we ordered four units of blood typed and crossed, and I told the nurses I was going to need help retracting to see adequately into the apex of the vagina. She called out of the room for any doctor to come help STAT in room 24.

Two physicians came immediately. They weren't my partners. They weren't close friends. In this time of litigious wildfire, they didn't have to come at all. But they did.

With better lighting and exposure, I could see that the patient had a vaginal side-wall tear that extended all the way up into the cervix and out of sight into the lower part of the uterus. This had occurred spontaneously—no forceps, no vacuum. It was rare, but there nonetheless. Her uterus began to firm up under the combined effects of the medications and continued massage, but the flow of blood continued.

She received those four units. And with the help of the other docs, we repaired her tear. Her recovery was unremarkable. But her gratitude was not. It was expressed in a plaque honoring her daughter's birth and thanking the physicians who had saved her life. It was also expressed with a sizable donation to the hospital.

Martha's next delivery was a scheduled cesarean because we were all nervous. The one after that was a VBAC (vaginal birth after c-section) because we were a little less nervous. Even then she had the complication of retained placenta due to a secondary lobe we were unaware of at delivery. Her final delivery was the one that begins this chapter—perfect.

All of Martha's children are miracles. All of them came long after the ruptured ectopic, which would have been fatal less than thirty years ago. The first child came only moments before what would surely have been another fatal event had the delivery not occurred in a modern hospital with skilled physicians in attendance. I will always be a part of this family, and I know that whatever I can do to help them in the future, I will go out of my way to do.

Sheila was twenty-eight years old at the time. A tiny woman, barely five feet tall, she had labored for twenty-two hours after induction because of toxemia. After pushing for three hours, we were forced to perform a cesarean. The baby was healthy. Mom did well. Everyone was happy until about thirty minutes later in the recovery room when her bleeding picked up markedly. She too was a victim of atony, or a uterus that failed to stay contracted and thus stem the flow of blood immediately after birth.

We returned to the operating room. I hurriedly discussed the situation with her very loving and concerned husband and received the expected instructions to do whatever was necessary. I assured him it would probably be easy to get a handle on. It was not. We tried direct massage of the uterus with the abdomen open, we directly injected it with the same type of medicines we had used systemically, we tried packing it, all to no avail. Reluctantly we proceeded with a hysterectomy while we transfused her with the first of what were to be more than eighteen units of blood. Believing her bleeding controlled, we closed after the hysterectomy. I had another talk with her husband, who was looking shell shocked by this time.

We were back ninety minutes later with bleeding from the vaginal cuff and the left pelvic side-wall. (Toxemia or preeclampsia leads to disorders in the coagulation system as well as fragile edematous tissues.) After another hour of surgery, we believed that all the bleeding was stopped that could be stopped. We left special packs in place and transferred her to the ICU, intubated and unconscious. Fifteen liters of salt water had made her extremely swollen and pale. I assured the husband once again that I thought we were over the hump.

One hour later we were back in the OR. I had called in a GYN oncologist familiar with bleeding dyscrasias as well as surgery in the deep pelvic side-wall. We worked for another two hours along with one of my partners, now also present at 2:00 a.m. It was all to no avail. We continued to transfuse her and could not stop the bleeding surgically. The tissue was too fragile, and vessels just ripped open when in contact with suture.

I was aware of a relatively new procedure from a conference out in California I had attended just two months before. One of the topics was uncontrollable pelvic side-wall hemorrhage. The procedure involved embolizing small pieces of foam into larger arteries with a catheter while under fluoroscopic guidance in radiology.

Faced with the imminent death of this new mother, we called in the only radiologist in town with experience in the area. We rapidly closed the patient and got her transported, multiple IVs, bladder catheter, endotracheal (breathing) tube, ventilator, and all to radiology. Over the next hour and a half, a new technology, the devotion of a skilled radiologist, and perseverence saved her life. It was truly a miracle!

Sheila continues to be one of my happiest patients. Always with a smile on her face, she revels in the constant joy of a growing son, and in seeing the sun rise each new day.

It was dedicated people in the middle of the night, it was continuing medical education, it was brand new technology that saved her life. I believe that dedication, education, and research and development may all be critically wounded by managed care. If that happens, another Sheila in the future will die.

I used to be a doctor. I spent my days and nights like I have described above. These cases were out of the ordinary, but every day, every physician involved in direct patient care does something that our parents would have deemed miraculous. For example, no matter what you believe the acceptable cesarean section rate should be, no one argues that in less than 5 to 10 percent of deliveries, it is lifesaving to mother and child.

What happened before the second decade of this century when the baby didn't fit? Well, midwives or doctors used instruments to destroy the fetal skull, if possible, and extract the fetus. If this wasn't possible, then hemorrhage, sepsis, exhaustion, and death for mother and child were inevitable.

How about ectopic pregnancy, until recently the number one cause of maternal deaths in this country? Now, most tubal pregnancies are caught early via radioimmunoassay blood analysis and vaginal ultrasound. We can treat the ectopic laparoscopically (telescope in the navel) with remote-controlled instruments, or more recently, even treat it with chemotherapy and avoid surgery altogether.

Doctors, aided by other medical personnel, perform lifesaving miracles every day. But now they tell me I'm a "health-care provider," not a miracle worker. What on earth are they talking about?

INTIMACIES

SOMETHING TRULY WONDERFUL can happen between a patient and her physician. When that special something "clicks" and you both know it's a good fit, the door opens to all sorts of ways in which the physician and the patient can help each other.

I've learned the value of trying to achieve the necessary sense of trust right from the first interview. It is that sense of trust that allows discussion of the most intimate details of a patient's life. These very private areas often include those which are causing her the most pain and distress.

"I can't believe I'm telling you this... I've never even talked out loud about this before." The young woman's voice was shaky as she dabbed at her eyes with the proffered Kleenex.

"You'll notice I have a box strategically placed in sixteen places in every room."

She laughed as she sat back in her chair and took a deep breath.

"I feel so stupid asking you about this when I hardly know you. I've wanted to talk about it for two years, but no one ever seemed like the right person to listen."

Dana crossed her arms over the purse in her lap, still clutching the wadded Kleenex. She was a strikingly beautiful twenty-eight-year-old woman with shoulder-length dark brown hair and penetrating blue eyes. She was "dressed for success" in a forest green suit and understated gold jewelry.

"Don't ever think your questions are stupid," I told her. "Ben Franklin, Madame Curie, and Thomas Edison were told that their questions were stupid, you know. Sex should be fun. It's healthy, it's a normal part of a loving relationship, and if you don't do something about the pain you've been having, it could destroy even the strongest relationship. You know it's no fun making love to a woman in pain. Men may be insensitive jerks a lot of the time, but even the dense ones know when you're having a good time and when you're not. If your lover knows he's hurting you, then he probably feels like an ax murderer every time!"

"Oh, he knows it hurts, but he's so gentle. We've tried everything. Different lubricants, different positions, I've been treated for yeast infections, bacterial infections, had my hormones tested, been off the pill, on the pill... nothing seems to help." Dana started to cry again, and I freshened her Kleenex from the box on the desk next to the picture of my kids and my dog.

"Now we don't make love at all. He's good about it, but, well, he's frustrated." I could hear the frustration in her voice as well.

"You may have noticed a fundamental principle of nature through all this, not applicable in every case of course, but still a good generalization," I said.

"What's that?" She looked up from her lap to me.

"Why, that men are horny 100 percent of the time! No matter how much he loves you, especially if you had the good sexual relationship that you described for the first two years, this problem will erode other aspects of your life together. So, we'll just have to fix it."

We spent the next thirty minutes during that first interview talking about possible causes for sudden onset of severe pain on insertion, after years of having no problem whatsoever with the same partner. Sometimes all it takes is intercourse during a severe yeast infection, or a brief period of inadequately lubricated intercourse, to develop a reflexive tightening of the strong muscles around the opening of the vagina. This is called "vaginismus." It is not under the patient's conscious control any more than the knee-jerk reflex.

We discussed the use of vaginal stents, or dilators, of successively larger diameter, held in place each night for fifteen to twenty minutes. If done over six weeks during which the patient is abstinent, this can completely cure the problem. We discussed other conditions more difficult to treat such as "vestibular adenitis," a viral infection of the tiny glands that surround the opening of the vagina or vestibule. The infection could be acquired sexually, and then rapidly lead to the scenario in which penetration was no longer tolerable. Its treatment would involve new concepts such as serial injection with interferon and possibly surgical reconstruction.

Dana left the first interview with new hope. True, she had to suffer through the brief biography I give to all new patients, supplemented by diplomas and pictures around the office, but I think openness about your own life and experiences fosters openness in the patient.

Dana and I started down a long road together that day. The sequential dilators failed. A laparoscopy did not reveal endometriosis or any other underlying cause for previous deep pain that could have in turn led to pain at the introitus. Sequential interferon injections over four weeks failed to relieve her pain, although they work 70 percent of the time. She almost lost her boyfriend at that point. Finally, four months after she started seeing me, we agreed to surgical excision of the affected area. She was scared and so was I. The surgery can leave scarring that could worsen things, if that were possible.

But it didn't. Her pain resolved completely when she resumed intercourse six weeks after surgery. She and her boyfriend got married, and I have since delivered a boy and a girl to the happy couple.

Restoring a young woman's sexuality is quite simply a wonderfully gratifying thing. It is in a very real sense saving a life as much as operating on an ectopic pregnancy, or performing an emergent cesarean section. Since my first successes at it, I have learned to probe for problems in this area of life that many patients are at first reticent to talk about. They're embarrassed and often think the problem is unique to them. Asking about it frankly, reassuring them that many people suffer from the same problems, often brings on a torrent of tears, but they're tears of relief.

Gynecologists do have a unique perspective on the doctor-patient relationship. Over 90 percent of health problems in women under age fifty involve their reproductive systems (both organs and hormones), or their breasts. Thus the very nature of our interaction with the patient is intimate, even without a word spoken. People are taught from age two that their genitals are their "privates" and most of them take it to heart.

But sexuality is not the only intimacy with which we deal. Women face problems with bowel and bladder function, infertility, weight loss, hair loss, mood swings, depression, bloating, breast tenderness, menstrual pain and/or heavy flow, and incredible stress with the triple role of wife, mom, and business executive. And unfortunately, in our society, women face the problem of battery and sexual abuse.

Sensitivity to these issues derives from a trusting physician-patient relationship that cannot be quantified. While some patients may tell me their intimate sexual problems at a first meeting, (my mom says that I just have the kind of face that invites people to pour stuff out) most save those discussions until they feel certain that I am empathic and can be trusted with a confidence. Often this comes after the delivery of a child. If you share what is arguably the most significant single event in a woman's life (and you're not a schmuck), she then lets you into a part of her that is reserved for very few. It provides an opportunity to offer help in ways that no stranger could. Knowledge of her relationship with her spouse and her children allows the physician to make the treatment decisions best suited to her life. This may be manifested in as simple an issue as choosing the right method of birth control, or as complicated an issue as how to best approach her depression.

All of you men reading this will understand one manifestation of this relationship. Try getting your wife to leave a gynecologist with whom she's comfortable because your company offers a PPO that doesn't include her doctor. It may seem irrational to you that she's willing to pay more per month to continue with her old doctor, but perhaps a woman places a different value than a man on having found someone with whom she can talk comfortably.

When I was a doctor, a trusting relationship was central to my successful interaction with every patient possible. As a healthcare provider, with annual patient exchange due to shifting contracts, limitations on my authority to make the right decisions by insurers, frustration and time wasted on paperwork and the phone, and an ever-worsening liability crisis, will I be caring for the patient with the same concern and compassion that I once could? You can decide after reading Part Three.

"TO PAINT A FINE PICTURE IS FAR MORE
IMPORTANT THAN TO SELL IT."
—EDWARD ALDEN JEWELL

PART THREE

HEALTHCARE PROVIDER: THE DEATH OF COMPASSION

THERE WAS A TIME not so very long ago when you could walk into any surgeons' lounge in the country and really learn something about medicine. As a resident in the early eighties, I remember rotating to the private hospitals in the Bay Area and learning as much or more in the lounge as I did in the operating room.

The reason was simple. Medicine was exciting. It was fun. People enjoyed what they did for a living, and they liked to talk about it. We knew our patients and cared deeply about new ways to help them. The potential benefits of a new procedure would be touted by one doctor and shot down by another. One doctor would have closed this way and another in a completely different way. Doctor X swore by this type of suture, another physician knew it was worthless for all the following reasons. Under normal circumstances, two doctors will debate about almost anything to do with medicine. Marshalling your arguments and championing the procedures that you feel hold the most merit is the process of medical education.

Walk into a surgeons' lounge today and you'll hear only two basic topics being discussed: managed care/health-care reform, and medical-legal issues. That's it. Period. I guarantee it. Outside of consultations, I haven't heard an honest discussion about how best to approach a patient's problem for probably three years.

Today, the frustration born of outside interference with diagnostic and treatment decision-making is so overwhelming that it occupies physicians almost to the exclusion of any other topics—with the exception of lawsuits. Medical-legal concerns are omnipresent, at least for those in my specialty. The American College of OB/GYN Survey in 1990 revealed that 77.6 percent of all OB/GYN physicians had been sued; the average number of claims filed against them was three. There is a 90 percent chance that an OB/GYN will be sued in his lifetime, so there's an excellent chance that several of the physicians in that lounge at any given moment are involved in the endless grind of ongoing litigation.

So the talk is of HMOs, PPOs, co-pays, precertification, quality assurance, value enhancement, capitation, deselection, Congress, preexisting conditions, etc., etc. We moan and gnash our teeth about malpractice premiums, letters of intent, depositions, expert witnesses, plaintiffs with spurious complaints, outrageous jury decisions and phenomenal awards, and losing our patients if insurance companies deselect us as providers. We swap horror stories of doctors facing financial ruin and despair. We share our fears about loss of retirement and the disruption of our children's education.

But there is no talk about medicine. None. There is no talk of the patients. Where is the compassion now? There is only concern with the self. And there is fear, fear so real you can smell it. I believe this to be a symptom of a very serious disease with a dismal prognosis unless we intervene immediately and forcefully. Doctors are becoming health-care providers by default. Our time, our efforts, our concentration, our energy, our emotions are being drained by these issues that do not have direct bearing on the improvement of our ability to care for the patient.

The following stories will give you a glimpse of the way in which managed care, coupled with a lack of tort reform, is unraveling our system by inexorably destroying what we once knew as the physician, and replacing him with a provider.

FRUSTRATION

As THE DECISION-MAKING POWER of your physician is stripped away, he is left powerless to do the right thing for your health. This alarming trend may have started with a little hesitation on the part of insurers to pay for everything with carte blanche, but it has escalated to the point at which poor decisions about your health are being made by uninformed individuals solely on the basis of cost. That means mounting frustration for doctors. And that, as we shall see, leads rapidly to danger for patients.

"Please continue holding. Your call is important to us. Do not hang up. Your call will be answered in the order in which it is received... "

I think I'd rather hear this disembodied, computer-generated voice over and over than return to the inevitable piano solo of "Feelings." But since the average time on hold can range from as little as two minutes to as long as forty minutes, there is usually ample opportunity to listen to both.

There was a time, they tell me, when a physician never had to speak to an insurance company representative on the phone. In fact there was a time when the physician's business office rarely spoke with an insurance company. It's not that there is anything particularly distasteful about speaking on the telephone. It is, however, difficult to do so for every single procedure, surgery, hospital admission, hospital stay, etc.

This time, after only seventeen minutes, a different voice comes over the speakerphone on the credenza behind my chair. I whirl around, snatching the handset from the cradle in time to hear...

"If you wish to inquire about a specific claim and you are a client, press the pound sign and one *now*. If you are inquiring about your premium or other account information, press the pound sign and two *now*. If you know the party's extension to which you wish to speak, press the pound sign and three *now*. If you are a physician, physician's office, hospital, imaging or surgery center, press the pound sign and four *now*. If you wish to continue holding, please press five, (God's honest truth— press five if I wish to continue holding) hold the line (again) and an operator will (may or may not) be with you soon... "

Like the puppet that I am, I press the pound sign and four.

"You have accessed the health-care provider client representative. If you wish to inquire about precertification for a procedure or admission, please press one *now*. If you wish to obtain a referral code number, press two *now*. If you wish to discuss reimbursement on a claim already filed, please press three *now*. If you need further assistance, please stay on the line and an operator will be with you soon."

I press one and pray that I'm almost out of the loop. After all, I do have three patients in the exam rooms. Since I'm scheduled in surgery during the insurer's lunch hour and their closing time is 5:00 p.m. EST, I must call between patients.

"Good afternoon, APSCO Insurance. Your health is our concern. Angela speaking. How may I help you?" Well, this is a start.

"This is Dr. Thurston in Dallas, and I'm calling... "

"Do you have the party's name to which you wish to speak?"

"No, I do not. As I was saying, this is Dr. Thurston and... "

"Patient name and group number please."

"The patient's name is Jackson, Brooke T., and I don't have the group number. Look I just need to speak to... "

"Hold, please," she commands, and I'm back to "Feelings" again.

Now, often this is where I get off. Patients are waiting. Some frontline person has already denied precertification for a medically necessary procedure, and I need to speak to the medical director. But this time I just can't hang up. The procedure is scheduled in two days. The patient informs me she was precertified with no problem, even had a confirmation number. My office staff was told the opposite on the same day. Dammit, I have to speak to somebody.

"I'm sorry, Doctor, but we have no Brooke D. Jackson. The group number would really help."

"It's T., Brooke T. Jackson, and I'm sure the group number would help, but that doesn't change the fact that I don't have it. Now all I need is... "

"No need to get testy now. Hold, please."

It's a good thing not everyone has video phones yet. When they do, I'm going to stop using the telephone completely. After fifteen seconds or so of a refreshing version of "People," Angela returns.

"I have it on screen now, Doctor. How can I help you?"

After an all-too-audible sigh, I try again.

"I need to speak to the medical director regarding the denied precertification on Ms. Jackson's laparoscopic ligamentopexy. The patient claims she was precertified, our office was informed that she was not."

"Well, let's see here. Nope. No record of either your office or the patient contacting us about this matter."

My intercom rings. It's my nurse: I've been on the line twenty minutes since the last patient checked out. Mrs. Schwartz is a postpartum and has her pediatrician's appointment in fifteen minutes all the way across town. Candy's crying in the treatment room with that right-side pain again. And Mrs...

"I'll be there as soon as I can."

"I'm in Hartford, sir."

"Oh, sorry, not you, that was the intercom, I've ah, ah, got people waiting. Look, I know the patient called. She was given a confirmation number. Here, it's on her chart. AP93-117493-22-018."

"Hold, please." Shit! Why does this surprise me every time? Even a fully orchestrated "To Sir, With Love" does little to placate me. After forty-five seconds or so, my misnamed Angel returns with good news and bad.

"Dr. Thornton?"

"It's Thurston, Dr. Thurston."

"Well, Dr. Thurston, we do show a Mrs. Jackson

receiving that number to precertify a laparoscopic tubal ligation, but after further review, and recognizing that her PPO policy does not cover birth control, we informed your office of the reversal and subsequent denial of her precertification."

"That would be just fine, except the procedure requested is a laparoscopic ligamentopexy for chronic dyspareunia."

"This procedure is for ICD9 623.8?"

"Could be, if that's the number for dyspareunia!"

"Well, painful sex is hardly a medical necessity, now is it?"

"I guess that would depend on your point of view. I would like to speak to the medical director, please."

"Have you tried lubricants? The computer under ICD9 623.9 lists dryness as the most common cause, you know."

"Ma'am, to be honest with you, I don't have the time or the inclination to discuss this with you. Now what is the medical director's name?"

"We don't give out our medical directors' names."

"Well, could you connect me with him now?"

"I'm sorry, that's quite impossible. We will give him the case number and ask him to call you back ASAP."

"Well, might that be this afternoon?" I queried hopefully.

"Most likely tomorrow. Our doctors are very busy, you know."

I wanted to say, "Is that so? Well, I have nothing to do but sit around and play this #@%$%^&*%^ game all day long!" But I just gave her the number for the OB office where I could be reached the following day.

Now, remembering how difficult it was to have made it this far, when a nurse retrieved me from an examining room the following afternoon for the medical director at APSCO's call, I rushed from the patient's room as though it were Ed McMahon on the line.

"Yeah, this is Dr. Thurston."

"Hello, I understand there is some confusion over Brooke Jackson's precertification?"

"Excuse me, but are you the medical director?" He sounded more like my great-grandfather.

"Yes, that's right, son." *Son?* Can you believe it? He

actually called me son. I wanted to address him as Dad, but thought better of it at the last second.

"Your name, please?"

"I am the medical director for this claim. My name is of no consequence. Now how can I help you, Doctor?" The emphasis on the last word established firmly what I had initially suspected. This guy was condescending to me, not vice versa! But if I was ever going to help my patient, I had to continue playing the game.

"My patient has suffered from deep dyspareunia for all of her adult sexual life. She has a severely retroverted, retroflexed uterus, and I believe deep penetration leads to contact with an entrapped ovary."

"Is that ICD9 623.8 or .9?"

Exasperated, I replied through clenched teeth. "I've been told it's 623.9. Does that help?"

"Hold on for a moment, please." Then came "Feelings" again. I was getting nauseous. I think this jerk was actually looking it up on the computer.

"Sorry about that. Listen, have you tried lubricants?"

"You cannot be serious. We have tried everything over the three years that she has been my patient. Her husband is cooperative but as frustrated as she is. It is beginning to seriously tax what is otherwise an apparently loving relationship."

"Well, what is it exactly that you propose to do?"

"As I said, a laparoscopic ligamentopexy."

"What is that?"

"What is what?"

"A laparoscopic liga... whatever you said."

"You're going to decide what procedure is medically necessary, and you don't know what the procedure is?"

"Now you listen to me, son. I was a general practitioner for fifty-five years in Flatbush, Nevada, and believe you me, I've done plenty of procedures, and many I'm sure before you were born, so don't talk down to me, Doctor!"

Stupefied, I actually apologized.

"I'm sorry, Dr.... er... sir, I only find it difficult to understand how you can make a decision in this case."

"Are you going to describe the procedure or not?"

"Yes, sure. It's a laparoscopic procedure in which the

round ligaments are redoubled and thus shortened, pulling the fundus to the anterior abdominal wall with only two small incisions. The ovaries are thus suspended away from the pouch of Douglas."

"Did you say suspended?"

"Yes. So?"

"That's procedure code G421.2. It's not covered. Any uterine suspension is considered elective major surgery, and it's not covered. Sorry."

"But that's the point, this procedure doesn't fall under the old code. It's outpatient. It takes maybe thirty minutes and the patient is home in two hours, back to work in three days!"

"Well, there's no code for it specifically. Furthermore, sexual enjoyment hardly seems a life or death matter, does it?"

"I don't think the patient would agree with you. Who else... "

"You can't talk to anyone else, Doctor. If Ms. Jackson wants this unnecessary procedure, she can pay for it herself! Good day!"

He hung up! He hung up on me! That was a twist. I usually hang up on "Feelings" or "People" or whatever.

That evening I called Mrs. Jackson and relayed her insurer's opinion. She had exactly no recourse, other than paying legal fees to sue an omnipotent insurance company that could well afford better representation than she. We agreed to talk again soon and try to come up with some other options. But I hung up knowing that the only real option was for her to live with her pain until after she had completed her childbearing and then pray for some pathology that her insurer would feel qualified her for hysterectomy.

Visualize this type of exchange happening thousands of times every day all over the country.

Similar exchanges occur between office personnel and insurance company R.N.s perhaps a hundred times more frequently. Frustration and wasted time are magnified by the fact that insurers use independent agencies on a contract basis to handle precertification. As a consequence, the potential for error in communication is increased, and the insurer has the opportunity (and frequently uses it) to deny payment retroactively, citing the nonbinding nature of approval before the fact by an outside agency.

In our OB office, we have about 800 ongoing pregnancies. Currently, our receptionist has to call for precertification for (1) OB care, (2), ultrasound, (3) oral glucose screening for gestational diabetes, (4) vaginal delivery or c-section, and (5) hospital admission. That is about 4,000 more phone calls than prior to managed care. Each of those phone calls can involve the "please hold" phenomenon for many minutes. Each of those phone calls is an opportunity for human error. Mind you, these 4,000 additional calls are for each of the patients with *no* problems. Additional calls are generated for anything not completely routine.

I am confident that any surgeon today could give you examples of the precertification nightmare. One of my colleagues recently carried on a conversation similar to the one I had above. It took over a week before he could actually talk to the "medical reviewer" for this particular company. After a long discussion about laser endometrial ablation it became clear to my associate that the reviewer had no idea what he was talking about.

When he repeatedly pressed the reviewer as to her qualifications, she couldn't give an answer to any questions about her internship, residency, practice experience, etc. After several more infuriating phone conversations, my associate discovered that the so-called "medical reviewer" was in fact a southern California medical student working on an hourly basis to help defray some of her living expenses. So a *student* made the decision that denied a patient a procedure that my colleague, with twenty years' experience and multiple board certifications, thought was appropriate.

I recently had precertification denied on a repeat cesarean section. I happen to be a big proponent of VBAC, or vaginal birth after cesarean. Educating the patient as to the safety of trying to deliver vaginally after a previous c-section has helped lower the repeat section and thus the total c-section rate. This in turn lowers length of stay, which lowers total cost.

That's all well and good. But VBAC is not appropriate for every clinical situation. The young lady whose precertification was denied had a 16cm posterior lower uterine segment fibroid (benign uterine tumor) blocking her birth canal. She also had a previous uterine rupture with an attempted VBAC elsewhere! Her insurer *still* denied payment for a scheduled cesarean section!

The patient had one anyway and paid the difference in hospital costs herself. But she was understandably indignant at what she viewed to be potentially dangerous strong-arm tactics to lower her hospitalization costs.

The frustrations are by no means confined to precertification. For the patient with painful intercourse, it is true, the insurance company's decision to deny the procedure may not be life-threatening, even if it leads to the dissolution of her marriage. It is also true that the decision with respect to the VBAC patient only cost her money and not her health. But other issues affect the welfare of the patient more immediately. In fact, other managed-care rulings—on length of stay, choice of pharmaceuticals, choice of laboratory tests, and restriction of appropriate consultation—are leading to dangerous situations.

OUTTA HERE

It has now become commonplace for patients to be discharged at the dictates of the payor without regard to their condition by people who lack an adequate understanding of the patients' needs.

Classic examples in the obstetric area would include patients seeking admission to the hospital for antepartum care due to high-risk conditions. These commonly include bleeding placenta previa, preterm labor, premature rupture of membranes, and preeclampsia or toxemia.

While it is true that in certain instances all of these situations might be managed with bedrest at home, each individual case is unique.

For instance, a thirty-one-week preterm-labor patient on a subcutaneous pump for administration of medicine might be managed at home with home monitoring *if* certain conditions were met. Those conditions might include proximity to the hospital, a cervical exam that was not worrisome with respect to dilitation, softness, position, effacement, and condition of the lower uterine segment, a vertex presentation, intact membranes, and others.

Now let's assume that, in this very common, uncomplicated circumstance, you have no idea what I am talking about. Now recognize that we may be seeking approval from an orthopedics nurse on the phone from Hartford, Connecticut, who has no more idea about the subtle difference in situations than you do. She makes the decision about whether the patient can stay in the hospital on the basis of criteria on a computer screen in front of her. Reasoning with her not only can require huge amounts of time, but is usually futile. If the patient is not independently wealthy and the screening nurse denies her stay, she's *outta here.*

So, let's say the patient lives 120 miles away, has a worrisome cervix, but is doing fine at this moment. Does she go home? Of course not, medically. But if her insurance denies her, the hospital wants payment. Even if she chooses to stay and can negotiate with the hospital, the uncovered portion of her bill can be astronomical.

Recently I had a patient two days post c-section with a 102.6 fever, a reddening, oozing wound, breast engorgement, anemia with a blood count of 24 (32 is normal post-op). Her insurance refused to pay for continued hospitalization despite IV, antibiotics, lack of bowel function, likely wound infection, and severe anemia with increased pulse and light-headedness.

She left the hospital after two hours of telephone work setting up and approving home care—IVs, nurses, etc. Admittedly, with cost-shifting on the hospital's part, each twenty-four hours would run an astonishing $1,800 including nursery care. At home the insurer paid only $900 per day. But this patient's care was altered solely on the basis of financial pressure. She was readmitted three days later with a severe post-op ileus (lack of bowel function), inability to urinate, continued fever, and a swollen arm from an infiltrated IV. She was in the hospital an additional five days. Was her early discharge either safe or cost-effective? Probably not.

NOT ON OUR LIST

Two weeks ago a patient of mine was diagnosed with a brain tumor of unclear etiology. While imaging studies showed characteristics compatible with a benign meningioma, the neurologist still recommended consultation with a neurosurgeon. The neurosurgeon with whom this neurologist works was not on the patient's PPO list, so he helped her choose one that was.

The approved neurosurgeon agreed that she needed surgery, but when they attempted to schedule it, they learned the hospital at which he operated was not on her PPO list. Appeals to her insurance bureaucracy have been fruitless to date. Surely this situation will be resolved, but if you were the patient, would you be happy spending three weeks working with administrative cretins?

This week a thirty-six-year-old woman, a longtime patient of mine, presented with gradually worsening left-sided pain. On ultrasound in the office she had a cystic and solid 11cm ovarian mass. I had delivered all three of her children. I had helped her through the tough times five years before when her mother had died of ovarian cancer. Now she needed me. She needed surgery, but I think she also needed me.

When we started to schedule her surgery, we discovered that she had been seeing me "out of network" for the last two years and paying out of her pocket for office visits. I told her I would do the surgery, and she could pay whatever she thought was fair over whatever time she needed.

That didn't solve the problem. The hospital I practice at was no longer on her network. Out-of-network payment to facility in this case was zero. Hospital costs would probably top six or seven thousand dollars. She and her firefighter husband just couldn't do it. So, with a newly diagnosed tumor and a history of her mother dying of ovarian cancer, she was forced to see a physician she had never seen before at another hospital.

NOT NECESSARY

Susan had just experienced her fourth consecutive miscarriage. Blood-testing of anti-cardiolipin, lupus anticoagulant, antinuclear antibody were all negative, as were X-rays of her uterine lining (HSG.) Every text in the world agreed that it was time for chromosomal testing of her and her husband. The karyotype on their blood samples would be $310 apiece. Her carrier, after multiple discussions with all my office personnel and finally after my discussion with the medical director, felt that this testing was unjustified. No appeal.

Corazon is a forty-two-year-old Latin patient with a history of previous tubal ligation. She has periods that last fifteen to forty days at a time that are unresponsive to hormonal treatment due to large uterine fibroids. Her blood count hovers around 25 (normal 40). She has bladder pressure and cramping almost daily. She was scheduled for a total abdominal hysterectomy. Her managed-care company said she would need a second opinion. I always welcome second opinions, but felt it absurd in this case and expressed this to the nurse reviewer. She said she would present it to the review board and let me know in two days.

True to her word, she called back in two days and told my nurse that a second opinion would not be necessary. Unfortunately, the reason was that they were denying the surgery outright. Had I tried hormonal therapy? We reviewed that with them again. Had I considered endometrial ablation? We explained why that was inappropriate. Had the patient ever needed blood transfusion? Well, not yet. We were instructed that when that was the case, her circumstances would be reviewed again. Bye. End of story.

DENIED... PREEXISTING

One of my personal favorite categories. As you are well aware, insurers, whether for life or health, frequently deny applicants coverage on the basis of preexisting conditions. This obviously applies to patients with chronic conditions, whether that be arthritis, lupus, psoriasis, etc. With respect to life insurance coverage, it is logical that a company would not want to pick someone up who already had leukemia, AIDS, lung cancer, or some other definitively terminal process.

But these conditions are not the ones that most frequently lead to a denial of insurance coverage. In fact, many of the conditions that lead to insurance denial the patient may not even have! Let me clarify this.

Recently a patient of mine was denied life insurance because in her chart, three years and two children before, there was a note about the patient inquiring after the safety of a certain antidepressant while having unprotected sex. She was told there would not be a problem. Now, she and her husband have applied for life insurance and been denied on the basis of that note. Well, not only was the patient not depressed, she never took the medicine. She had asked the question for her next-door neighbor! I never prescribed the drug, there is no evidence that I did so, and yet after multiple communiqués and documentation, the insurer will not reconsider.

Another common one for health insurance is HSV, or genital herpes. It is estimated that 10–20 million American women have this viral infection. We now know it *is not* the precursor to cervical cancer. It has no long-term health effects. It may not even be necessary to do c-sections for active lesions in the near future, as we have come to realize that only first-time lesions hold high risk of infection for the newborn. Despite these facts, I constantly receive notification that a woman's health insurance with a new carrier has either excluded *any* problems with her reproductive tract or denied her coverage completely, solely on the basis of a history of genital herpes.

Now here's the real kicker. I have patients in whom we have suspected genital HSV, cultured for it, had it return negative, never have another suspicious episode, and *still* be denied! I have patients with recurrent abnormal Pap smears for whom we have performed an office cone biopsy or LEEP procedure, removed the tissue in question, had Pathology confirm the *absence* of true dysplasia, or precancerous change, and *still* they are denied coverage in the future.

Preexisting conditions have become a convenient,

often undocumented mechanism for insurers to deny coverage of entire portions of a person's health care, like their reproductive tract. Whether it's HSV and denial of maternity benefits, or fibrocystic breast changes and subsequent denial of coverage for a totally unrelated breast cancer, current carte blanche with respect to the insurors' ability to deny coverage prospectively as well as retrospectively, adds significantly to the frustrations of health care for both physician and patient.

The stories of wasted time and thwarted effort from any practitioner in this country are endless. "Frustration" no longer adequately describes the feelings of many. Some physicians would prefer a completely socialized system to this, where at least there would be only one payor—the government—to deal with, and that payor would at least be somewhat responsible to the voters. Insurance companies, by contrast, are responsible only to stockholders—and stockholders want *profits*.

MENTAL ANGUISH

OUR LITIGATION NIGHTMARE has extended to all industries and all walks of life. It is devouring our nation's productivity and making us less competitive on the world market. There's not much relief in sight because our legislatures are full of attorneys, many of whom make a good living from personal injury litigation. The Clinton Administration bill proposed in the fall of 1993 would have *removed* caps on mental anguish that are now in place in some states.

While our litigation crisis increases malpractice premiums, drives the spread of costly defensive medicine practices, and undermines trust in physicians as a whole, it has a more insidious, destructive effect as it eats away at the joy of practicing medicine. Soon, there will be no reason to risk everything, everyday, for anybody.

Until near the end of my residency in 1985, I honestly thought "torts" were something that you ate, rather than vice versa. I now recognize that the food has an "e" on the end, and the legal term deals with a civil litigation in which the defendant physician may in fact be consumed. The litigation crisis may not be news to anyone, but the way in which it directly affects your health care might be.

We live in a society being destroyed by the erosion of individual responsibility. Consider:

• The wayward teen who rapes or murders or steals or sells drugs is now viewed as the unfortunate victim of societal circumstance. Somehow we have let them down, and so their behavior is less reprehensible.

• When a three-year-old gets run over by a truck at 11:00 p.m., it's no longer the parents who are responsible, but clearly the maker of the insufficiently bright luminescent paint on the tricycle that failed to adequately protect the child.

134

• When a patient smokes cigarettes for forty years and gets lung cancer, it's not his responsibility, but the manufacturer's for inadequately warning him during the first twenty years of his habit.

• When a woman gets breast cancer, it's not just bad luck, bad genes, and/or her failure to follow recommendations of breast self-exam and mammography that are responsible for the stage of disease at discovery, No, the last physician she saw is responsible for failing to diagnose her.

We have all heard the absurd stories of litigation brought by criminals falling through skylights, or grossly obese people "emotionally injured" by a restaurant lacking seating in which they could comfortably fit. But these suits could not be brought in the absence of liberal juries who view large corporations as well-insured, deserving targets; magistrates who permit the filing of totally unfounded actions that defy common sense; and people willing to fill the role of plaintiff to get rich out of someone else's misfortune.

Medicine is only the very visible tip of the iceberg. The litigation crisis is undermining this country's productivity and siphoning its lifeblood into the coffers of large, flourishing law firms. Corporate funds go in increasing amounts to defend frivolous suits. Many of the USA's largest pharmaceutical companies have moved overseas to avoid the huge legal costs of headquartering in the United States.

While corporations are affected by legal fees and costly product alterations undertaken to avoid litigation, medicine is affected both directly and indirectly as well. Obviously, rising costs of malpractice coverage can and are passed on to consumers, but this represents only the most minor effect on medicine.

I believe there are three major mechanisms by which the litigation crisis directly influences the quality of your health care: First, costly defensive medicine practices; second, the creation of a quandary for the managed-care physician who is losing decision-making authority; and third, the creation of a state of mind in your physician that is incompatible with optimum functioning.

The Clinton Administration estimated $6 billion in defensive medicine costs for 1994. The American Medical Association estimated $100 billion. My guess is that any estimate you pick is too low. Defensive medicine practices are so ingrained that they are not even consciously recognized as such. Much of the preoperative, admission, and antenatal testing done currently as routine could be completely eliminated from a purely medical standpoint. But in a society where perfect outcomes are not just expected but *demanded*—or else—these expenditures will continue.

If you walk into the emergency room tomorrow night and tell them you have the worst headache you've ever had in your life, you won't get out of there for less than $2,000. Now the likelihood of you having a malignant astrocytoma is extremely small. A full physical exam including blood pressure, eyes, ears, and neurologic exam would be adequate to diagnose your headache on a preliminary basis. Then you would be discharged to see how things progressed with some pain medication in the next twelve to twenty-four hours.

Sounds simple, but that won't happen. Instead, unless you flat out refuse, you will get a CAT scan and/or an MRI and, in all probability, a lumbar puncture. Even if you refuse, you'll be asked to sign a form saying you left against medical advice. The ER doc just can't take the one-in-a-thousand chance that you're the one with the tumor.

Let's take an example closer to home for a gynecologist. Other than hearing of a worrisome finding on her mammogram, there are probably no words a woman dreads more than, "Your Pap came back abnormal." Ever since Georges Papanicalaeu designed the screening test for cervical cancer in the 1920s, an abnormal finding has been synonymous with possible precancerous disease of the cervix. Some of the mystery surrounding this particular killer has been resolved with the recognition of the causative role played by the sexually transmitted HPV virus. Those individuals who are virginal, celibate, or monogamous can now be reassured that they are at lower risk. But just as we achieve a better understanding, defensive medicine rears its ugly head in an unexpected way.

This is America! If a woman gets cervical cancer, she makes three calls: her husband, her mother, and her attorney. Plaintiffs' attorneys have become increasingly savvy. They know that "abnormal" is a broad term that encompasses cells on a slide that may have nothing to do with precancerous changes and that such cells can be found on almost half of all Paps. The vagina is full of bacteria. The uterus is sterile. Since the cervix connects the two, it is, by definition, full of inflammatory cells. These inflammatory cells can mimic very, very early precancerous cells.

So, if an unfortunate young woman gets invasive cervical cancer, an expert witness is paid to find any abnormal cell on a slide five years ago that was reported as "normal," and the corporation that owns the pathology lab can just shell out $10–20 million regardless of the patient's treatment and prognosis.

Naturally, the nation's pathologists have moved to protect themselves from the rising tide of litigation. Instead of reading only 3 percent of Paps as abnormal, with another 25 percent labelled "normal, but with inflammatory atypia or reactive change," now they read about 30 percent as "abnormal" but with the same commentary. In short, the new Bethesda Classification for Paps, in place since late 1992, was developed in large part to protect pathologists from frivolous litigation. I'm all for that, except for one tiny little problem. There are human beings at the other end of these newly inflated abnormal Pap rates. Guess who gets to call them with those frightening words?

The current recommendation from the American College of OB/GYN is to re-Pap all nonprecancerous abnormals in three to six months, at the same time performing more extensive testing with colposcopy (fancy binoculars) and biopsy, if indicated.[1] Sounds logical, but it's cold comfort to the terrified patient who wants to know why she can't come back *tomorrow*, if not sooner, for a repeat. (Cells take months to turn over, inflammation can be treated, etc.) Colposcopy is expensive and time-consuming as well. Furthermore, with liability shifted so neatly to the gynecologist, many of them are simply choosing to grossly overtreat with expensive office laser or electrical excisional procedures.

So once again, external forces come into play to warp the physician's judgment to the detriment of the patient. Defensive medicine costs are underestimated due to just such scenarios as this. Their contribution to spiraling costs is not always as upfront as doing an MRI for a headache.

One more example. Let's suppose that you have a pregnant patient who's scared of ultrasound, or even better, an insurance company who won't pay for it. In any event, the patient doesn't get an ultrasound exam at any point in pregnancy and the baby is subsequently born with an ultrasound identifiable defect, such as spina bifida, or tetralogy of Fallot (a common heart defect), or short-limbed dwarfism. If you haven't thoroughly documented the reason you didn't *insist* on an ultrasound exam and specifically mention the need to rule out this disease, then you're in deep you know what.

Let's expand this point to include our second harmful effect of overlitigation, the quandary of the physician in managed care. Let's suppose the patient's managed choice HMO does not pay for routine ultrasound. Furthermore, let's suppose that this Kroger checkout girl is not just loaded with cash. When her baby has an obvious spina bifida that was sono diagnosable, do you think the insurance company becomes the defendant? No way. The insurer can only be held liable for the original cost of the claim. After all, the insurer told her they wouldn't *pay* for a sonogram, not that she couldn't have one! It was the *physician* who should have told her how important it was to a safe outcome.

Physicians in a myriad of managed-care scenarios are being forced to make suboptimal-care decisions by insurers, but are then held accountable for anything other than a perfect outcome. If they make the appropriate diagnostic decisions, it will either cost the patient out of her pocket, or, as in many networks where patients are not allowed to pay for any services beyond the approved ones, it will have to be done at no charge. If the physician knuckles under and allows the insurer to dictate to him,

138

then there will be no sympathetic defense when a potentially diagnosable defect shows up. It is a no-win situation for patient and physician.

Finally, the current litigation crisis causes a huge number of formerly effective physicians to simply deteriorate due to their own "mental anguish." While mental anguish is usually a term used to describe the nonfinancial damages suffered by a plaintiff from a wrongful action, it could equally be applied to the state of the defendant physician's thought processes.

Physicians are human, and their state of mind is reflected in their performance. For the most part, physicians also have a tremendous sense of responsibility, or they wouldn't spend eight to twelve years of their lives working literally minimum wage for 120 hours a week in order to learn how best to help you.

Now let's superimpose onto this sense of responsibility the accusation that some specific act of omission or commission harmed a patient. Every physician is familiar with the Hippocratic credo, *Primum non nocere*—First, do no harm. If in fact one lives his professional life by this medical golden rule, what do you suppose the psychological repercussions of such an accusation might be? I suppose it would be somewhat like telling Captain Picard or Captain Kirk that they purposefully flouted the prime directive.

Never mind whether a mistake was actually made or not, and of course in medicine that question is often open to interpretation. What would be the repercussions of such an accusation on an honest, dedicated physician? I can tell you. I've been there. Imagine how you would feel if you received a card in the mail from an angry parent who tells you she can't tolerate the thought that *your* children are healthy while her child is not.

Mental anguish is the answer. It comes in all forms and it camps at your mental doorstep for a very long time indeed. First there is the self-doubt, the self-questioning. Could I have done better? Did I really make the error I am accused of, and if so, did it really lead to the outcome? Did I do something, even inadvertently, that hurt or injured or killed my patient?

Doctors ask themselves these questions all the time. They're asked in the shower, they're asked on the highway, they're asked while tossing and turning and trying to sleep, they're asked when their kids are trying to get their attention, they're asked while ignoring your spouse's need for comfort or support, they're asked while seeing an office patient who brings the topic to mind, they're asked while they're operating, or sitting in church, or singing in the choir, or while they're supposed to be teaching Sunday school.

They're asked when they're supposed to be relaxing out to dinner, or a movie, or a cocktail party. They're asked while they throw a ball to their dog, or mow the lawn, or while they're apologizing to their wife for the hundredth time because they didn't hear what she said. These questions go round and round and round in their head's sometimes for months at a time. They preoccupy them after a tragic outcome while waiting for the possible suit. They hang over them after notification of a suit to be filed in ninety days. They vex them before, during, and after depositions. They hunt them down before and after trial or settlement.

And don't let me kid you, these aren't the only questions. Because even if you're eventually convinced that your action or inaction did not lead to the poor outcome, there are questions in your mind about your *own* outcome.

What will this do to the most important thing I have, my reputation? What if I lose everything I've saved for my kids and my wife? What if the case comes to trial and we get a jury so empathic with the plight of the plaintiff that the medical facts are ignored and they find a judgment against me for more than my insurance limits? Do I declare bankruptcy? I wonder what's involved with that? Can they attach my wages forever so that *I'll never get through this?*

There are new dangers as well. As the National Data Bank, which records malpractice suit information, is made public, physicians may be deselected from HMO and PPO provider panels on the basis of one settlement. Already proposed National Quality Assurance Data would eliminate providers with *one* case settled for $30,000 or more in the last five years. This will preselect providers who are younger and less experienced. Further, it will penalize the patients of thousands of excellent physicians who settled cases out of court rather than endure the torture of years of litigation, even if the issue was one of legitimate clinical judgment.

In many states, including Texas, a single anonymous complaint to the Board of Medical Examiners can launch an investigation in which *one* instance determined to represent "substandard care" (i.e., *one* error in clinical judgment established retrospectively from an adverse outcome) can encumber your license to practice medicine. In a managed-care environment, even a former slap on the wrist, such as mandatory CME (continuing medical education) for a brief period, can cause a physician to be removed from HMO provider panels. If, say, 70 percent of his patients are managed care, that slap on the wrist amounts to the same thing as revocation of his license!

Imagine going to work every day in a situation in which there is *zero* tolerance for error. In short, despite being human, you are simply not permitted to make a mistake, or it may cost you everything you have in the world.

It's ridiculous. But that's what the American physician lives with every day. In an instant-gratification society, a society that sees miraculous new high technology every day, the concept of a bad outcome has become unacceptable. If things don't turn out the way they're expected to, somebody's responsible, and somebody must pay.

Well, somebody is paying, and it's not the physician, it's the patient.

You're paying because your doctor is forced to do things that are medically unnecessary so that he can try to protect himself.

You're paying because your doctor is being forced into a situation in which someone else really makes the medical decisions under the guise of deciding what will be covered, and yet the doctor retains the liability.

You're paying because your doctor is dealing with

emotions and stresses that shouldn't be there and that affect his judgment and performance in a very real way.

So what can be done?

There are some simple answers. The rest of the civilized world, from Japan to Germany, has figured it out. First, make the plaintiff pay all costs if he or she loses. That will seriously limit frivolous suits.

Second, don't allow contingency fees. Force lawyers to work like everyone else, for a fee. In legitimate cases the damages then go where they belong, to the plaintiff.

Third, limit awards for pain and suffering. If there can be no price on intangibles, don't let juries or judges put absurdly high ones in place.

Fourth, allow juries to know about alternate compensation. In many states, the plaintiff (unbeknownst to the jury) may already be a millionaire due to compensation from other settlements or insurance payouts. When a jury is instructed to extrapolate lost wages for the estimated working lifetime of the plaintiff, compensation of the injured party from another codefendant for the same claim is superfluous. In other words, lost income should only be calculated once, then split among the defendants, not paid out over and over by each defendant.

The litigation crisis has now taken a back seat to the shifting paradigm in which the physician's decision-making power is being eroded. But just because it's in the back seat doesn't mean it's not still there when you reach your destination. And there are new dangers as well. The new breed of health-care provider may be employed by a big HMO corporation. His malpractice premiums may be paid as part of his compensation. As he adopts the casual attitude of the shift worker, coming to work at nine and leaving at five, seeing rotating patients every day, he may not go that little extra mile to ensure the best outcome. After all, he's only one of many physicians who may care for a particular patient. It's not like he's solely responsible for your health anyway.

Besides, who ya gonna sue? The corporation, where the deep pockets are. I just work here, lady.* (See "Notes")

DANGER

MANAGED CARE, WHETHER "MANAGED" by an insurance industry intent on profit or by the federal government intent on a misguided, misconceived notion of guaranteed comprehensive health care for everyone is fraught with danger. There ain't no free lunch.

Our legislators' moral imperative—to provide health care for everyone—has run up against simple economics: somebody has to pay. In order for the insurance companies or the government to guarantee that their proposed paradigms will function, they must obtain control of as many variables as possible. They must control both providers and patients, and in the government's case, misguided egalitarianism may lead to equally rationed mediocre care for all of us.

And the mediocre care would come at tremendous cost financially. (The "Clinton plan" would have cost a trillion dollars in new spending over the next eight years, according to the Congressional Budget Office.) The cost in quality would be tremendous, with millions of people forced into plans they don't want and which would restrict their choices and undermine their doctors' ability to make decisions.

With the failure of the Clinton health-care reform effort in the fall of 1994, the future of reform is anything but clear. But I want to show you how changes already wrought by managed care are affecting you daily. Institutionalizing these changes by law simply hastens the destruction of the entire system, a destruction already well on its way.

"Katie, you know where my patient is by any chance?" I continued to randomly flip over, turn around, and otherwise mess up charts in the rack and on the nurses' desk.

"Twy in twelve, Docta. You wememba, the pelvic woom?" The no-nonsense head nurse of the graveyard shift in the emergency room swept around the corner with a pen clenched in her teeth, an IV and angiocath in one hand, and a liter of saline in the other.

"Oh, you mean just like always for the last nine years?" I asked innocently as Katie rocketed down the hallway towards a trauma room. She glanced back over her shoulder and hollered, somewhat impeded by her oral grasp of the Bic, "How do you ewer fine your own socks, Docta?"

I picked the metal clipboard out of the plexiglass slot marked "12" and glanced over it as I walked quickly down the gray linoleum hall. Without looking up, I negotiated the gurneys and wheelchairs much as a trained Marine would a familiar obstacle course. The various conveyances held the usual assortment of disoriented elderly, inebriated, and lacerated street people, screaming children with everything from ear infections to broken limbs, as well as anxious, overweight people in their sixties, oxygen masks in place, worrying about heart attacks.

At the end of the hall, I turned right to a cul-de-sac with three exam rooms. All were designated as "female" rooms, purportedly because they contained the necessary equipment considered the stock and trade of my specialty. Tonight, the door to "11" stood open. A youngish redhead with an IV in her arm sat on the end of the bed, vomiting into a trash can held by an unhappy male who had his head turned to the side. The sound of her heaving was overwhelming, unstoppable, like a diesel truck shifting gears on a steep grade. I said a brief silent prayer of thanks that this was not my patient, since I am one of those empathic vomiters who simply cannot be in the same room with an upchucker.

I pushed open the door to "12" and immediately saw that Suzanne Rogers was not in a good way. She had called earlier in the day, complaining of severe abdominal pain. A nurse had told her that since she was on the pill, her last period was on time, and her pain was on her left, that it probably wasn't anything serious—maybe a muscle strain or something. But the pain kept getting worse, so I had asked them to meet me at the hospital.

Now Suzanne lay on her right side, knees curled up and moaning. Her hospital gown was soaked with sweat. Her dishwater-blonde hair lay limply across her face. Her eyes, half-open, focused only after I spoke. "Fancy meeting you here at one-thirty in the morning! Couldn't sleep either?" My quip brought only the weakest of smiles to her face.

"Hi, Dr. T! Am I glad to see you! Nobody around here seems to take me seriously." Each word was pseudo-whispered, as if the breath required for normal volume was too painful to contemplate. Her husband sat nervously fidgeting on the edge of a plastic chair at the foot of the bed, his arm outstretched to rub her foot.

"There's something bad wrong with her, Doc," he said. "These folks here say it's just a ruptured cyst, but I don't know. She don't look right to me. Never been a time she didn't read a story to one of the kids at bedtime, and I did 'em both tonight while she soaked in the tub. It just got worse after that. Then she started throwin' up, and moanin' and carryin' on, and I got scared."

Suzanne had been my patient for at least six years. I delivered both their six-year-old daughter and their four-year-old son. She was not a powder puff. Both her deliveries had been unmedicated, and her performance had been as perfect as Katerina Witt skating to her second gold medal. Her husband was right. For her to look like this, something bad was going on.

Gently, I helped her roll onto her back. I listened to the total silence in all four quadrants of her belly where bowel sounds should have been. Just tapping on her lower tummy, especially the left, brought a wince and a yelp of agony. There was no doubt, something was causing a peritonitis. A ruptured appendix? Less likely with pain starting on the left and then spreading, but still never lower than third on the list of possibilities. Could have been a ruptured cyst as the intern had suggested to them, but you don't often get cysts on the birth control pill, and besides, Suzanne just looked too sick.

I took her pulse at the wrist. One hundred twenty-two! Pretty far up there to be sustained by pain alone. The sweating and the pallor all fit with the onset of shock secondary to intraabdominal bleeding. In the absence of a ruptured spleen caused by a direct blow, ectopic pregnancy had to be number one on the list. I asked her a few more questions about her history and got all the information I needed from her and her husband.

"You're gonna be all right, kiddo," I told her. "We'll get you something for pain, I'll check some lab results, and I'll be right back." I stroked my hand over her sweat-soaked brow and gave her husband a wink for reassurance.

Once outside, I called the OR and told them to get ready for possible laparoscopy, but more probably an emergency laparotomy for a ruptured ectopic pregnancy. They said they'd alert anesthesia for me. I collared the intern whose name was on the chart as he came out of the X-ray reading room behind the desk. After brief introductions, I told him I had some quick questions about the lady in room twelve.

"Oh, the ruptured cyst?"

"You got the adjective correct, but I believe the noun incorrect."

His look was somewhere between incredulity and annoyance.

"Look, it's 2:00 a.m., just spell it out."

"You took that lady's history, didn't you?" He admitted that he had, in addition to doing a very painful pelvic exam.

"What's the first thing you always ask any male ER patient over the age of eighteen?" The intern had no problem with that one. He responded as we all could from rote, "Are you now, or have you ever been, in the service of any branch of the armed forces of the United States?" Even if the man was in a drunken stupor, an affirmative answer would get him an ambulance ride to the nearest V.A. hospital.

"Now, what's the first thing you ask any girl or woman over the age of twelve who presents with abdominal pain?"

He knew that one too. "When was your last period? But I asked her that. It was right on time and a pill

146

withdrawal at that. She's had no irregular bleeding, not even spotting, and she's never missed a pill by her story." The intern seemed a little smug at his success so far.

"What kind of pill is she on?"

"I didn't ask. So what?"

"What other meds is she on?"

"I guess I didn't ask." A little less smug now.

"Well, I'll tell you... Katie, call the lab and add a serum pregnancy test to twelve's lab, STAT will ya? And keep a nurse in there all the time for the next few minutes. Oh, and open up her IV, and type and cross her for four units... Now, where were we?"

"Other meds."

"Oh yes. She was supposed to be on a 1/50 pill because of her anti-convulsant meds and their interference with estrogen metabolism."

"Oops. I guess she wasn't, huh?" The intern looked a little like a puppy who's just spotted the rolled-up newspaper in your hand.

"Here's the part you're gonna love. Her HMO refused to pay for that brand of pills. They have only three brands on their formulary, so they substituted a generic 1/35 when she got her three-month supply of pills in the mail. She questioned the color change on the phone to the pharmacy, but they assured her the insurer would only have substituted a generic equivalent. Incidentally, it's illegal to do that in this state unless I specifically allow substitution, which I wouldn't have in her case. I'll bet you dollars to donuts she's bleeding like a stuck pig inside from a ruptured left ectopic pregnancy."

"Well, let me know what you find, and ah, thanks." The intern shuffled to the rack and grabbed the next chart. It seemed like only yesterday that I lived in his twilight world of near-total sleeplessness.

Needless to say, Suzanne had to have her left tube removed. If we'd caught it earlier we might have saved it, but without knowing she was pregnant, Suzanne hadn't been in for any early testing.

There are three separate ways in which managed care could have killed Suzanne Rogers.

First, the obviously inappropriate and illegal

substitution of a nonequivalent prescription drug in the interests of cost-cutting.

Second, had Suzanne been forced to see a physician unfamiliar with her history of pain tolerance with natural childbirth, the doctor might not have held a high enough index of suspicion of an intraabdominal catastrophe. He might also have missed her history of anticonvulsant use and not thought to actually check on the identity of her oral contraceptive.

Third, even had Suzanne suspected a pregnancy, under a managed-care plan she would have had to waste time seeing her designated internist "primary care provider" before being allowed to see her OB/GYN. As it was, her insurance company—unbelievably—*denied payment* for her ruptured ectopic retroactively, claiming that she bypassed her primary care provider in not seeing him earlier in her pregnancy. The fact that she was unaware of her pregnancy did not sway them, nor that the operation was life-saving and emergent. The outpatient surgery cost them well over $6,000, less than a third of which was physicians' fees. As far as I know, the patient and her husband, a dairy farmer, are still fighting the good fight with her insurer.

Such stories abound. Recently a patient of mine was driven to my office at 4:00 p.m. on a Friday. She was bleeding heavily, cramping severely, and believing she was in the midst of a miscarriage. After looking at her card, my receptionist informed her that she should be aware that her insurer required her to see her primary care provider first or they would deny pregnancy-related claims.

The patient, despite her misery, called the 800 number from the lobby. She got an operator in Connecticut who told her there were no available appointments for ten days with her acceptable providers. After she patiently explained the emergent nature of the problem, they looked up an alternative M.D. on the computer and told her a network doctor in Winnsboro (one hundred miles east of Dallas) could see her in half an hour. She told them unless they wanted to pay for a Life-Flight helicopter, it seemed unlikely that she'd be able to get there!

But (insane) rules are rules. It was the only option they would provide. I saw the patient in the office for nothing. She required a D&C, which the hospital allowed her to pay off over time.

Many managed-care plans now require women to get an authorization from their "primary care provider" in the form of a referral number before they can see their OB/GYN. Recently a twenty-nine-year-old patient of mine called her "managed choice" PCP, who just happened to be a woman internist located forty-six miles from where she lives and works. She asked for a referral number to be allowed to see me, her OB/GYN of six years, for a new-onset mid-cycle bleeding and pain with intercourse. She was denied by the internist's office, being informed that she had already received one authorization only two months previously.

The fact that the previous referral was to an ophthalmologist for an eye infection, they claimed had no relevance. My patient reluctantly acquiesced and made the trek to see the internist.

When the patient called me, hysterical, in tears, later that afternoon, she related an unfortunately all too common scenario. The internist had painfully inserted the speculum and examined her vagina for six minutes. When apparently unable to visualize the cervix, she asked my patient if she'd had a hysterectomy! My patient, somewhat taken aback, replied that she had not. Was something wrong? The internist proceeded with a bimanual pelvic exam and told her that she also couldn't feel her ovaries. The errors were compounded by subsequent statements about my patient's potential for infertility problems due to her abnormal anatomy, questions about her husband's fidelity in light of her pain and bleeding, cultures for sexually transmitted diseases, and blood tests for suspected hormonal abnormalities.

All of this was baloney. The bleeding was caused by a problem rectified by changing her pill. The pain was caused by the most common type of vaginal infection other than yeast, easily treated with a cream. Her anatomy was totally normal, as later documented in my office with vaginal sonography at no cost to put her mind at ease.

For women under fifty, 90 percent of health-care needs involve the reproductive organs, breasts, or reproductive hormones. Internists get six *weeks* of training in this area, while your OB/GYN has four to six *years*. Should women be denied access to their OB/GYNs in a misguided, unproven attempt at cost containment? What about gynecology procedures like colposcopy to follow up abnormal Paps, electrosurgical and laser cone biopsies of the cervix, hysteroscopy to see into the uterus, endometrial biopsies, Depo-Provera birth control injections, Norplant placement and removal, IUD placement and removal, and even birth control pill management with over sixty pills on the market with eleven different progestins in all different ratios to multiple different doses of estrogen? Internists and family practitioners in different parts of the country have assumed all of these responsibilities with little or no training under the auspices of restrictive HMOs mandating gatekeeper systems that do not designate the OB/GYN as the provider of women's health care.

In 1994, 30 percent of all HMOs did not allow a woman self-referral to her own gynecologist.[2] Furthermore, "capitated" systems, which we'll examine more closely shortly, financially penalize the family practitioner or internist for referring to the specialist, OB/GYN or otherwise. HMOs may argue this as cost effective and "preventive medicine," but much data suggests otherwise.

According to the National Ambulatory Medical Care Survey in 1990, annual exams by gynecologists were twice as likely to include a Pap smear, three times as likely to include a pelvic exam, and twice as likely to include a breast exam. Competence aside, if the internist or family practitioner is too busy to even perform a complete physical that includes the parts of the woman's body most likely to harbor dangerous disorders, is it good preventive medicine even if someone can show a cost savings?

And could you be expected to show a true savings in the long run when accounting for delayed diagnosis and consequent increased expense for breast, cervical, uterine, and ovarian cancers? What about early diagnosis of ectopic pregnancy before rupture, endometriosis, or ovarian tumors?

By the same token, does it make sense for an OB/GYN to manage difficult cardiac arrhythmias, complex endocrinopathies, or for that matter, surgical problems outside his area of expertise, such as neuro, cardiac, or orthopedic surgery? Of course not.

I have a question for you husbands out there who advocate a restrictive HMO because it saves you a couple of hundred dollars in the next year, even though it doesn't permit your wife to see her gynecologist. Would you let her get on an airliner flown by a pilot who you knew had only six weeks' experience flying Piper Cubs before he stepped into the cockpit of the 767?

The U.S. House of Representatives passed a 1994 resolution "expressing the sense of the House... that OB/GYNs should be designated as primary care providers for women in Federal laws relating to the provision of health care." Delaware, Georgia, and Virginia have passed similar resolutions. California passed a law in September 1994 requiring payers to consider OB/GYNs primary care providers. Maryland and New York have passed laws that require payers to allow women direct access to their OB/GYNs for at least one visit per year.[3] But still most states have no such protections for women's access to their OB/GYNs.

Many managed-care plans now require their patients to get referrals from their PCP for each OB visit during their pregnancy. Furthermore, my office staff needs an average of five different precertification codes for just a vaginal delivery, all requiring separate phone exchanges throughout the pregnancy. Failure to follow the rules of each insurer, which literally change daily, can result in nonpayment.

But the dangers are not in any way limited to restrictions on availability. Cost containment by an outside agency that does not have the patient's welfare as its primary concern can have a direct negative effect on outcome.

Case in point: Just this week one of my patients delivered twins at twenty-nine weeks, three months early.

During the previous three weeks, I had carried on no less than five phone conversations with her insurer. In the final call two weeks ago, I was again denied approval for home monitoring on the basis that the patient had not already been hospitalized and treated for preterm labor.

The whole point in the management of twins, of course, is prevention. Multiple gestation starts out as high risk for preterm delivery by definition. Once preterm labor begins, it may be impossible to stop, but home monitoring of uterine contractions with telephone transmission of the tracings may identify the process early enough for treatment to be effective. Even much cheaper daily phone contact with a nurse might head off preterm delivery.

The cost to the insurer would have been $150 per day for the monitor, or even less for daily nursing contact. That may seem like a lot until you consider the *$3,500 a day* they will pay for at least the next fifty-five to sixty days of NICU care. You may note that comes to around $210,000! Well, here is reform at work! This is certainly "value enhancement!"

If my patient had been able to follow my recommendation without the interference of her insurance bureaucracy, not only might she have saved the system huge expense, she might have had her twins go home with her instead of spend weeks on ventilators. With the excellent (but costly) care they will receive from the Neonatal Intensive Care Unit, they stand a good chance of not developing the chronic pulmonary, renal, intestinal, and hearing problems frequently associated with the premature, but only time will tell.

Two years ago a forty-eight-year-old patient of mine was in for a yearly exam. Since her mother and an aunt had both died of ovarian cancer, I recommended she have a screening blood test called a CA-125. Even though the test is only 80 percent sensitive, any help in early diagnosis is worthwhile. Only later did I discover that when she was told at the front desk that the $125 test would not be covered by her HMO, she elected to forego it.

You know where this is going. Fourteen months later when she returned slightly late for her annual exam, I found a left ovarian mass. This was confirmed by office ultrasound, and subsequently her CA-125 was found to be extremely high. Her disease had spread throughout her abdominal cavity, dooming her to both the discomforts of chemo and radiotherapy and the certain prognosis of death on the very near horizon. Now, no one can say that her disease was confined to one ovary (curable by removal of the ovary) fourteen months before, or even that her CA-125 would have been positive. But if both of these things were true, her care would have been much cheaper, and, oh yes, she'd be alive.

On any given day, I can now ask any physician colleague who is in active practice to recount the managed-care nightmare he experienced that *same day*! Today, for instance, I passed through the lounge on the way from a surgery to the locker room and heard two doctor acquaintances exchanging stories from earlier in the same day. One had been denied approval on a blood test to determine whether a woman was carrying the gene for Duchenne's muscular dystrophy.

The patient's brother had DMD and her sister was a carrier of the X-linked recessive disorder. She was aware of a 50 percent chance that she carried the gene on one of her X chromosomes. If she was a carrier, then because any son of hers would get one of her X chromosomes, he would have a 50 percent chance of having the disease. And any daughter would have a 50 percent risk of being a carrier. However, if she did not carry the gene, her progeny's risk was zero.

Without carrier-testing, the couple faced the 50 percent possibility of their child either carrying the gene or, in fact, having the disease, with that discoverable only at amniocentesis. Then they would be faced with the choice of terminating their pregnancy or risking a life-shortening, debilitating disease through a son, or potentially passing on the disease in a daughter. Therefore, carrier-testing to determine her status was appropriate.

Appropriate to her doctor, that is. The medical director of the insurance company, on final appeal, stated that the test was not medically necessary. The medical director went on to say that as far as he was concerned, "reproduction itself is not medically necessary." (An

153

interesting viewpoint and I suppose defensible on an individual basis, but hard to accept from a species perspective.)

The other physician had just been denied the use of heparin, the only blood thinner shown to be safe in pregnancy, for a woman who had nearly died with a massive pulmonary embolus in her last pregnancy. The insurance reviewer refused to pay for the medicine because it was not on their OB formulary. She suggested instead a drug that is strictly contraindicated and shown to cause severe birth defects in humans. Once this was pointed out, she simply responded that the medicine was not covered and that the "client" could foot the $1,500 bill herself if she wouldn't use their formulary choice.

Danger. There is demonstrable danger in removing health-care decisions from the hands of patients and their physicians. Decisions about diagnosis and treatment should be dictated by the patient's needs and not by fiscal considerations. These decisions should not be dictated by forcing patients to gatekeepers or designated primary care providers; by forced referral patterns or lack thereof with respect to specialists; by misguided, ill-informed purse-string management of pharmaceuticals; or by restricting diagnostic laboratory and imaging tests thought necessary by the attending physician.

Ill-informed purse-string management is not confined to the private sector. Recently the National Cancer Institute changed their recommendations for screening mammograms to start only at age fifty, overruling their own National Cancer Advisory Board.[4] They did so largely after reviewing computer analysis of multiple studies, including one roundly criticized Canadian study which concluded that survival time was not increased in women under fifty.[5-10] No other group bought into the study. Not the American Cancer Society, not the American College of Surgeons, not the American College of OB/ GYN, not the American College of Radiology. Only the federally funded NCI came up with a recommendation that would save the government hundreds of millions should national health insurance come to pass.

The Colorado Mammogram Advocacy Program (CMAP)

has recorded the findings of every single mammogram performed in the state for a number of years. Guess what? More cancers were diagnosed in the forty to fifty age group than the fifty to sixty age group. In fact, about 30 percent of all the breast cancers detected were in women under fifty.[11] Our own data at Presbyterian Hospital in Dallas corroborates this. Out of 27,249 mammograms performed since 1992, 234 patients were diagnosed with cancer. There were seventy breast cancers in women under fifty, or about 30 percent!

Follow the NCI's recommendation, and a huge number of these women would have been diagnosed at a later stage and grade and consequently with a worsened prognosis.[12] All of the major societies have stuck with first mammogram at thirty-five to forty, with at least every other year from forty to fifty, and yearly from fifty on. But many insurance companies seem to like the National Cancer Institute's recommendations. All of a sudden, some insurers aren't covering mammograms for women in their forties. Even if it's true that $2 million are expended to save every life under fifty, who would society benefit more from saving, the forty-two-year-old working mother of small children or the seventy-year-old grandmother in questionable health?[13]

Danger. Let a respected institution like NCI be influenced largely by cost concerns and not solely by health concerns, and people are going to die needlessly. For twenty years we've worked to make women aware of the importance of mammography, and in one controversial move, the NCI may have done irreparable damage to women, and possibly fatal damage to some young women.

But the danger inherent in these scenarios is nothing compared to that looming on the horizon in many parts of the country and in fact already the case in other parts. By that I mean the danger of the institutionally employed physician, in which the institution is the contracting entity with employers and insurers.

Traditionally, or at least since World War II, insurers have contracted with individuals to cover some percentage of their health-care costs after a deductible is met. As costs have risen, this paradigm has shifted such that employers contract with insurers, and the employee-patient is then directed to a PPO plan (preferred provider) with little or no deductible and a tiny co-pay such as five to ten dollars.

The preferred providers aren't "preferred" in the traditional sense, of course; that is to say, they're not chosen because they are known to practice good medicine, but only because they've signed a contract to accept reduced fees in exchange for listing. Both hospitals and doctors play this game. All of the dangers enumerated above can rear their heads in this situation, but at least the physician is still autonomous, even if the patients' choices of doctors, drugs, and hospitals are channeled.

But things can get worse. Then comes "capitation." An ugly word for an ugly idea. Capitation is simply a per capita system. An insurer will pay a contracting entity, let's say for sake of argument a hospital, a set amount per patient per month to cover all eventualities. Any money left over at the end of the fiscal year is profit for the hospital. If the hospital either employs, or by nature of the capitation contracts, substantially controls the physicians on its staff, their compensation too is tied to funds left over at the end of the year. The physician's individual productivity in dollars is tracked by computer and broken down into "fixed overhead" such as rent, utilities, insurance, etc., and "variable overhead" such as supplies, laboratory tests, imaging tests, consults with specialists, and hospitalizations.

It's easy to see what happens here. A system comes into being in which both doctors and hospitals are rewarded for delivering *less* health care. Not better, not necessarily more efficient, but *less* health care. A financial incentive—in fact, for the patient, a life and death financial incentive—is created to lower costs at all costs.

Recently I had lunch with the medical director of a nearby family practice group. They in fact had formed their own HMO without walls and took almost 90 percent of their patients on capitation. During the usual tuna salad and iced tea fare in the hospital's conference room,

I asked this sixty-year-old physician how his group handled referrals.

"What do you mean, referrals?"

"I mean, if a patient presents with a difficult arrhythmia and you want them to see a cardiologist, do you subcontract that out or what?"

"We don't do that." He said it with finality.

"You don't do what?" I said, thoroughly confused.

"We don't refer. To anyone. Ever."

"You mean you handle renal failure without a nephrologist, and seizure disorders without a neurologist, and ruptured discs without a surgeon?" I was incredulous.

"Exactly."

"Is that a good idea? I mean are your patients really getting the best care?"

"Who said anything about the best care? That's not the game anymore, Doctor. The bottom line is the game. There are twelve family practitioners in the group. We'd love to have your guys be our obstetrics arm. Currently that's the *only* thing we sub out."

"But what if you just don't have the expertise to handle someone's problem? What if it's life-threatening?"

He looked at me with what I can only describe as contempt. Wiping the mayonnaise off his chin and throwing his napkin on the plate, he abruptly pushed back his chair and stood up.

"I guess the patients should have thought about that when they bought cheap insurance!"

You'll be happy to know that we didn't join their merry little band. When I related this story to my brother, the heart surgeon, he laughed bitterly.

"My partner had a bitch of a month in June," he said. "Three out of six of his coronary bypass patients died either in or right after surgery. He was devastated. But not everybody was unhappy. The first week in July, he got a certificate in the mail for being the "low cost provider" in cardiovascular surgery for the month of June!

"It's the God's honest truth!" he went on. "Even got a write-up in the HMO paper. Of course no one mentioned that ICU time is *very* expensive, and if your patients die on the table, it's extremely cost-effective!"

This is Danger with a capital D. At least in a one-party payor socialized system, there's no *disincentive* for care. Sure, the government might totally screw things up and end up rationing health care in a big way; but at least under such a system the hospitals and doctors aren't *paid* to underdiagnose and undertreat you.

It is true that various forms of managed care have successfully reduced health-care costs for many large companies. But the outcome data for these changes in terms of patient satisfaction and overall quality of care is embryonic.

ACADEMIC MEDICINE

THERE IS ANOTHER DANGER not to be underestimated. All medical schools depend on their urban medical center institutions as training grounds for medical students, interns, and residents. These academic centers associated with medical schools are also the central nervous system of the country's medical research. Our institutions of higher learning in medical education are being seriously threatened by managed care.

Teaching hospitals must now compete with nonacademic institutions for the exploding number of managed-care contract patients. They are being forced to negotiate rock-bottom prices for services, often below cost. As managed care sweeps the nation, both HMOs and hospitals are acquiring outpatient-care facilities, physicians' practices, nursing homes, laboratories, etc., in an effort to ensure they are not left out of the market. As Dr. Jerome Kassirer points out, academic medical centers and managed-care plans have very different missions.

"Managed care organizations, particularly those owned by investors, are required only to apply existing knowledge to routine patient care. Academic medical centers, on the other hand, create new knowledge, develop and assess new technologies, evaluate new drugs, educate medical students, train tomorrow's physicians, and care for the sickest patients."[14] Dr. Kassirer goes on to show that the costs of these programs, combined with demographics of patient populations, make the costs for these academic institutions 30 to 40 percent higher than the cost for competing proprietary or community hospitals. Managed care organizations, with an eye solely to cost, avoid academic institutions for their patients. As a result, many such hospitals are left over-bedded, underused, and in real danger.

If we undermine our nation's capacity to do basic research while at the same time diminishing our capacity to educate physicians, we will poison our own future. There is genuine reason to be alarmed at what profit-driven managed-care organizations may do to our academic institutions, albeit indirectly, and thus what they may do to our children's and grandchildren's healthcare.

We should continue to look for solutions to cost-containment issues that do not dismantle our current medical infrastructure and put obstacles in the way of what trained physicians know to be the optimum medical choices. At the same time, we must strive to avoid destroying our world-class academic institutions in the rush to hold down costs. The danger signs are proliferating, and it is time to take action.

"LET US NOT LOOK BACK IN ANGER,
OR FORWARD IN FEAR, BUT AROUND
US IN AWARENESS."
—JAMES THURBER

PART FOUR

RESTORING COMPASSION: IDEAS

DON'T GET EXCITED NOW. Don't go kiddin' yourself. The health-care crisis is not going to dissipate under the influence of my startling intellect over the next several paragraphs. However, I would like to make what I feel to be a few valid observations and point us in a direction that stands the best chance of attaining health-care reform without eliminating the best aspects of our current system.

What do we want? That's pretty easy. We want to keep our relationships with our doctors, and let our doctors keep making the decisions about our care. But we want to halt the upward spiral of costs associated with the delivery of our health care, while maintaining quality and at the same time improving access to the system for all income levels. Simple, right?

Before we can fix anything, a rudimentary understanding of what went wrong seems important. I believe there are five basic forces that have combined to leave us in this mess, and we shall examine each one briefly.

THE PROBLEMS:

INSURANCE

FIRST, INSURANCE. Who are we kidding, here? Last year over 85 percent of claims filed were for less than one hundred dollars! We now expect insurance to pay for everything, including routine preventative care. I can promise you that in the immediate postwar (The Big One—WWII) period, when companies first began offering health benefits in lieu of higher salaries for all sorts of tax reasons, they did not envision the Frankenstein's monster to which they gave birth.

The insurance industry drives health-care costs skyward in two basic ways. One is obvious, the other not so blatant. The first, of course, is profit. Hey, this is America. I don't begrudge them profit. Bidness is bidness! But when you ask the average American to give you a dollar figure for his annual health-care costs, what does he give you? Not the cost, but the *insurance premiums he pays*. Well, news flash, that ain't the cost. The insurance industry has successfully decoupled actual health-care costs from patients' pocket books. All of us know that *if you've met your deductible,* and you show up in the ER with a migraine, and they say, "Maybe we ought to do an MRI scan for $1,400," you say, "Go for it!"

As we shall see in more detail, as traditional indemnity plans are supplanted by preferred provider organizations (PPOs), and more recently multiple variations of health maintenance organizations (HMOs), deductibles have been greatly reduced or even eliminated with the patient paying only a token co-pay at the point of service. So insurance companies increase costs directly by increasing premiums to maintain profit, and indirectly by encouraging usership. Increased usership increases total health-care costs, although it may damage an individual HMO's profits. Thus, usership is becoming subject to insurer control as well, as we have discussed earlier with respect to "gatekeepers."

HMOs are apparently getting a handle on this variable,

however, because as of January 1995, the nation's four largest HMOs posted liquid assets of greater than $1 billion apiece. As of December 1994, according to the *Wall Street Journal*, six midsized HMOs were sitting on roughly $500 million dollars. These liquid assets accrued at greater than 15 percent for many HMO firms in 1994. Wall Street analysts are now kept busy just trying to guess where the giants will put their excess cash next!

Despite HMOs' claims of promoting sweeping cost savings in the delivery of health care, these savings may be often realized by the HMOs, not the consumer corporations who contract with them. In general, those profits are not passed on to stockholders, either. For the most part they're being used to acquire larger and larger shares of the health-care market.

MEDICARE/MEDICAID

Next, Medicare/Medicaid. Our well meaning, socially progressive, paternalistic, early sixties' federal government decided that it should be the keeper of the elderly and the downtrodden. You remember, the same government that brought you the well-oiled piece of machinery called "welfare!" Well, great idea, guys, but a few problems have arisen. From fraud, to incompetence, to underfunding, coupled with poor management, to all the problems associated with any massive top-heavy bureaucracy, Medicare/Medicaid illustrates the federal government's inability to manage an unimaginably complex social issue. But in the last decade, Medicare/Medicaid's contribution to rising health-care costs has been directly attributable to their *decreasing compensation for services.*

While this decrease in compensation is supposed to help lower costs, it has the opposite effect by driving cost-shifting to private insurers across the board. And what do they do in turn? Bingo! Raise premiums. Where do you think the $37.50 Tylenol pill came from? Are the hospitals just gouging you? Maybe a little, but mostly not. In many states, private institutions are forced by law to care for all indigents who walk in the door. You're already paying for their health care at your neighborhood state/county facility, but many of our state legislatures, in a politically correct dedication to egalitarianism, have mandated that the indigent *have a right* to the same quality health care that you working stiffs do.

If we as a society decide that health care is a *right* and not a *desire*, then we have the *obligation* to ensure that said health care is delivered. If we impose that obligation on the federal government, it will be empowered to use its sweeping authority to ensure that the right to health care is enforced equally. It can and will tax you without recourse, it can and will require any confidential information it sees fit, it can and will regulate any facet of the medical industrial complex, it can and will determine which approved plan you may participate in, and it *can and will* decide who you may choose as your doctor.

I submit that despite our benevolent intent as members of society to provide for the less fortunate, *health care is not a right, but a privilege.* We may strive through private charity, through personal voluntarism, through our organized religious outlets, even through some government entitlement, to provide health care for the less fortunate. But to declare health care a *right* mandates absolute equality of deliverance and eliminates the role of the very free market forces that built our current system into the envy of the world.

The single party payor system, i.e. the federal government as insurer, has been proposed to meet this obligation. Many other forms of government-controlled managed competition have been set forth as well. But even without any of these changes, you currently get to pay three times for health care. You pay with federal taxes for Medicare, state taxes for Medicaid, state and local taxes for county facilities, and you pay for higher insurance premiums brought on by the aforementioned laws guaranteeing indigent care at private facilities, coupled with decreasing Medicare/Medicaid payouts which drive cost-shifting.

THE PROBLEMS

DEFENSIVE MEDICINE

Number three on the hit parade is defensive medicine. The Clinton Administration offered $35 billion as an annual estimate for excess cost related to this issue. The AMA estimated well over $100 billion, a number I feel to be much closer to the truth. In truth, any number you pick is probably low.

Let's go back to your postdeductible migraine headache. When the doc offers you an MRI or CAT scan *after* your normal neurologic and fundoscopic (eye) exam corroborated by your normal blood pressure, is he doing it because he has nothing else to offer? No. Prior to about 1978, he would have offered you calm reassurance, two Percodan, and told you to call him in the morning if not better. And you know what? You would have left happy, and cared for, and a whole lot sooner than you would leave today.

Today, however, the ER doc has to consider the one in a gazillion chance that you have a brain tumor, or aneurysm, or subdural hematoma, or etc., etc. Because God forbid, if you did have one of those and he missed it, it could cost him his career, his retirement, his children's education, his life savings, his self-esteem. Little things like that. Don't get me wrong. I'm not suggesting that he shouldn't look for those things *eventually, if symptoms persist,* just that he doesn't have to look right then, when you may never have symptoms again!

Defensive medicine is now so ingrained that it's literally a bad habit. Doctors don't even realize it when they're doing it. Take preoperative lab work. Often hundreds and thousands of dollars are spent on testing to uncover incredibly rare abnormalities that (might) lead to (potential) problems with anesthesia or surgery, most of which could be handled at the time if in fact the (near mythical) problem ever actually came to be.

Other societies from western Europe to Japan are flabbergasted at the percentage of GNP we pour down the drain for defensive medicine, for insurance to cover product liability, and for product modification to avoid problems that were once avoided by good parenting! Wake up, America! Tort reform on a national scale is long, long overdue.

NEW TECHNOLOGY

The fourth big contender propelling medical costs skyward is clearly new technology. Couple this with defensive medicine, along with competing hospitals in the same geographic area, and you have the prescription for logarithmic cost increases.

There is much validity to the belief that humanity has progressed more technologically in the last twenty years than it has in the preceding 80,000! Digitalized, base 2, instantaneous information transfer coupled with the millions of intricate pathway options provided by interlinked computer chips has quite literally changed our world. Advances in laser technology, fiber optics, and robotics have given us further modalities with which to apply the awesome power of our computers. While MRI may allow imaging quality never before possible, and Gamma knife may allow neurosurgery without an incision, the technologies involved are quite disparate. There is one similarity, though. They're expensive. Big time expensive! Millions of the little green guys! And if hospital "A" wants to take patients from hospital "B," which happens to have a new MRI located only three miles away, they may feel they have to have their own MRI or lose the revenue those patients will generate. Well, the General Electrics of this world didn't just fall off the turnip truck, so they raise their prices in this scenario, not lower them. Thus competition for high tech drives costs *up*, not down.

Where does the hospital get this kind of huge revenue? Why from cost-shifting of course! (See above.) Who pays for that? You do, via increased premiums. The need for expensive equipment and procedures, remember, is not just driven by hospital competition, but by defensive medicine practices as well. Thus the pressure to have the most advanced capabilities is intense, and your bill (read: your insurer's bill) will reflect it.

We should also note that technology has increased costs in a more subtle way, through the proliferation of specialists. In the 1930s, only 20 percent of physicians were considered specialists. Insurance paid only for hospital care, and specialists required higher out-of-pocket payment than general practitioners. In the 1940s, specialists were given higher rank and higher salaries by the military. Many GPs then sought specialty training under the GI bill. In the 1950s, with federal grants for research on the rise, most of the money went to specialists, who dominated evolving medical schools. By 1969, 50 percent of doctors were specialty boarded. By 1990, 66 percent were specialists, and only 14 percent of medical students were entering primary care residencies.[15]

So historically, better pay fueled the natural tendency to specialize in a society in which the medical-legal environment demanded perfection and the average student couldn't possibly keep pace with the technological advances in every field of medicine.

INFLATION

Lastly, there's our old friend inflation. So now it's only 4 percent, big deal! Now figure out what 4 percent of $150,000,000,000 is. I'll tell ya, it's a bunch. $4,500,000,000, or $4.5 billion. That's inflation's contribution annually to our estimate of defensive medicine costs. Ouch! As Harry Truman once said, "A billion here, a billion there, and pretty soon you're talking about real money."

THE SOLUTION:
MANAGED
COMPETITION ???

CONTRARY TO POPULAR BELIEF, understanding managed competition is not humanly possible. It may be defined, as we did earlier, as a health-care delivery system in which decisions about diagnosis and treatment are made not by the people trained to do so, but by people working for profit-motivated corporations. It is a term that encompasses a myriad of paradigms for the entire medico-industrial complex, many of which have little similarity to each other. But one thing is clear, managed competition involves a radical departure from our current system of third-party payors, free choice of doctor and facility, and government care of the indigent through county facilities funded by Medicaid.

There is a common thread, however. Most of the scenarios involve the insurance companies becoming the providers themselves, either by owning hospital systems and the affiliated physicians' practices, or by controlling delivery through a capitated system, in which the insurer pays a group of physicians or a hospital-run corporation a certain number of dollars per patient (employee) per month for any and all care provided (i.e., per capita). The physicians are then compensated from the pool of money *left over* at the end of each fiscal quarter. Most of these scenarios call for "gatekeeper" primary care physicians as described earlier. Well, guess what? Do you think this primary-care-provider-(family practice, internist, pediatrician) driven system is going to allow referrals to specialists for many problems? For any problems? Not when it costs them their livelihood.

With a capitated system, doctors will be given a strong financial incentive to avoid expensive tests and referrals because those tests and referrals would diminish their personal income. Well, you say, that's the idea, right? We want to cut costs, don't we? No, remember the goal:

We want to cut costs, increase access, *and* maintain quality health care. The assumption that the specialists we've trained over the last thirty years are now superfluous is patently absurd! Medicine has become so complex and changes so rapidly that it's difficult to keep up with your own area of expertise from week to week, much less everyone else's area as well! There is no way that quality of care can remain unaltered if the least-trained physicians (in terms of years of residency) in our system are suddenly called upon to diagnose and treat conditions for which they may have little or no training, and on top of that, are paid *not* to refer to specialists who will be more knowledgeable about diagnosis and treatment of specific conditions. Under a capitated system of managed care you will get a very different health-care product, don't kid yourself.

Initially, when HMOs further decoupled health-care costs from the consumer's pocketbook with only small co-pays at the point of service, usership skyrocketed. But many fledgling HMOs have failed, because a co-pay of five or ten dollars or nothing gives the patient *no disincentive* whatsoever for going to the doctor for the slightest problem. As usership has risen, so have costs. But many managed care companies and their parent insurers have found new ways to counter this trend by actually limiting number of visits permitted per year, whether to emergency rooms, primary providers, or specialists.

As alluded to already, the nation's top ten HMOs each have liquid assets of $500 million to $2.6 billion. Many HMOs have financial positions so strong that the insurance boards of several states are beginning to question and sometimes deny rate increases.

Doctors and hospitals are being squeezed by HMOs to do their jobs more cheaply or risk losing portions of their patient population. And while they are doing their jobs more cheaply, HMOs literally have so much cash that they don't know what to do with it. HMOs in general do not provide for or own the medical infrastructure; thus, their overhead—primarily administrative, legal, and advertising costs—is low. No wonder the *Wall Street*

Journal dubbed these HMOs "money machines" in December of 1994.

In essence, managed care has already created a system to which every criticism of the defunct Clinton Health Care Plan applies; i.e., bureaucrats make the decisions about your care, not the doctors who are trained to do so; patients are restricted or forbidden to choose their own doctors; health care *is* being rationed through capitated primary care providers; and the entire medical system answers not to its patients, but to America's gigantic and powerful insurance industry.

It would be false to imply that all the changes wrought by managed care have been negative. Companies like Columbia/HCA Health Care with its 308 hospitals and 125 outpatient facilities nationwide have forced efficiency on competing hospitals.[16] Not unlike Wal-Mart in its phenomenal growth spurred by cost-cutting efficiency, Columbia/HCA is literally calling the shots in many areas. Their ability to buy fixed overhead items in bulk allows them to consistently underbid area competitors for HMO contracts. Many of their competitors have had no choice than to become leaner. Often this means forming alliances with area facilities that used to be considered competitors or face absorption or even closure.

Columbia has also made innovative moves like installing computer software, which improves physician efficiency by automating lab results, patient databases, and pharmaceutical information.

Nevertheless, this rising giant represents the epitome of corporate medicine. While its leadership favors tort reform and eliminating preexisting conditions, it sees no place for the nonprofit community hospital. Its hospitals are under corporate chain of command, and when the word comes down from on high, that's the way it is. The traditional board of trustees, made up of community-minded philanthropists, has no real place in this system. Like it or not, beneficent or not, efficient or not, corporate medicine's goal is to improve the bottom line.

Assets for Columbia/HCA have risen from $200 million in 1991 to $15 billion in 1994, or roughly 75-fold.[17] It's a given that their profits continue to rise as well. That's great for the stockholders, probably good for the economy, but will only be good for the patient if the ability to choose her own physician is preserved and the physician is allowed to determine the course of her care. Such growth based on efficiency would be expected to pass savings on to businesses.

In fact, managed care *has* significantly reduced health-care costs for many large corporations. According to a survey by the employee benefits consulting firm, Foster Higgins, of over 2,400 employers, over a third were able to halt or reduce their company's rising health benefits tab in fiscal 1993. They did so by putting the squeeze on doctors and hospitals. They provided financial incentive to steer employees into restrictive managed care plans and used their leverage to gain price concessions in a competitive marketplace.[18]

Xerox contracted with 204 HMOs nationwide in 1993. Employees were given the option of traditional indemnity coverage at much higher rates, and only about 30 percent chose to make the financial sacrifice necessary to maintain their freedom of choice. The other 70 percent of employees were given choices between different HMOs, thus forcing the HMOs to compete for Xerox premium dollars.[19]

GTE admits that they would like to force their 94,000 U.S. employees into even more restrictive plans. As is, they kept their rate increase on the average health benefits plan to only 1 percent in 1993 versus the national average of 8 percent.

The fastest growing type of plan however, is the "opt-out" plan where employees are given the option to pay more out of pocket to retain their choice of physician. DuPont's long-term strategy includes such plans for its 66,000 employees and 75,000 retirees.

At the end of 1993, 27 percent of employees nationwide were in a PPO plan allowing some degree of choice, 19 percent were in restrictive HMO "gatekeeper" plans, and 7 percent were in "opt-out" combinations. The remaining 47 percent were in some type of more traditional indemnity plan.[20]

So, all forms of managed competition will tend to

provide "less" medicine with respect to possibly needed tests and referrals and be forced to combat higher usership with restrictions on access. It seems clear that managed care can and does lower costs of health care. But does it maintain the quality that we agreed at the outset was the other portion of our goal for reform? Is that "quality" quantifiable in a way that employers as purchasers of health care can really use? Even if companies shell out millions to consultants to evaluate length of stay, referral patterns, mortality rates, prescribing patterns, test fees, and office visit charges, can they accurately assess, for example, the feeling a woman needs to have about her OB/GYN after she's just been up in the stirrups for a very personal problem? Can they accurately assess the value of the extra phone call at home to check on her after her surgery, or the hand held tightly while an anxious patient goes to sleep knowing you'll take good care of her, or the kind of relationship where a hug is natural and a true comfort in the face of bad news?

The vice-president of marketing for one of the fastest growing insurance providers in Texas said in an interview recently, "What they [the public] perceive as high quality is not really quality at all." The implication is that Aetna, MetLife, Sanus, PruCare, Cigna, Humana, etc., know what is high quality, and in their paternalistic beneficence will make those decisions for you!"[21] Already insurers are eliminating or "deselecting" the physicians who cost them the most money. The ones who remain on their network will be the ones who deliver the cheapest health care. The definition of "quality" used to be the care that led to the best outcome. Not anymore. The vice-president of health services management for a large Texas insurer has said that, "Quality medicine is cost-effective medicine."[22] Evidently, the old adage, "You get what you pay for!" applies in all walks of life, except medicine.

Proponents of managed care say the new system will impose discipline on physicians who were formerly guided by only their own avarice. The exact opposite is actually the case. The autonomous private physician makes referrals, orders CAT scans, etc., when he deems them appropriate. There is no financial incentive for these decisions except

174

for the few who abused lab ownership, which has been largely curtailed by Congress's Stark legislation. On the contrary, the HMO physician must allow finances to play a role in his decisions. Under the new paradigm, every diagnostic test, every referral, every expensive treatment adversely affects his personal income.

In most insurance-owned HMO systems in which the managed care company contracts directly with the employer, and then the HMO contracts with providers such as hospitals, surgi-centers, and physicians, who has the motivation to meet the patients' needs? The hospital strives to please its customer, the HMO; the HMO wants only to please its customer, the corporate employer. Who wants to please the patient? If the physician has large portions of his patients contracted from the HMO, or worse, if he has an exclusive arrangement, where must he place his first allegiance? When the interests of the HMO and those of the individual patient clash, how will the contract physician prioritize? When the physician is faced with "deselection," the very loss of his patients because of practices not deemed adequately cost-effective by the HMO, will his decisions not be tainted? *Who then is motivated to put the needs of the patient above all else? The answer is simple and regrettable. The answer is no one.*

Managed competition succeeds in devaluing the physician-patient relationship to near nonexistence. Don't delude yourself when you hear different systems promise you "choice." They mean you may select from a limited list of providers with whom they have contracted. These contracts are never for more than a year, so you could be forced to change providers annually. Already we see patients who, having been with our practice for ten years, develop a condition requiring surgery (major hospital expense) and be forced to seek another physician and hospital because we're no longer on their network.

Who cares, you might ask? You may forget that physicians are people too. I may strive to give the same care to everyone who crosses the threshold of my office, but I know it doesn't happen. If I've delivered all four of a woman's children and feel a part of their family, I go to extraordinary efforts to keep her happy and well. Not

175

to mention that the patient's comfort level with her physician dictates her openness and willingness to provide an accurate history of what might be an intimate or embarrassing problem. Medical history is still 95 percent of the diagnostic process, and an inadequate history because of patient discomfort or time constraints, leads to errors in judgment.

So, managed competition might decrease costs, but won't appreciably increase access, grossly restricts the patient's own authority to make choices for herself, decreases the level of care in terms of technology and expertise, and undermines the physician-patient relationship.

SOME ANSWERS

As previously intimated, neither I nor anyone else has the answers on how to put out the firestorm of controversy surrounding health care in this country. But many of us have suggestions about how to at least avoid suffocating in the foam from our own extinguishers.

INSURANCE

First, we must restore the link between *actual* costs and patient payment. If a third party pays the bill for anything, you're going to buy more than if you're footing it yourself. There have been many proposals about how to deal with this phenomenon. I believe the most logical would include medical IRAs or so-called medical savings accounts (MSAs) set up by employers or, alternatively, the government. If it is true that the *average annual cost* of health care to the family of four is less than $1,500, then something close to this amount could be withheld (approximately $120/month) and placed in an interest-bearing investment account. Routine visits to the doctor would not involve any insurance claims or even significant paperwork. The charges would be handled electronically by debit card drawn on your MSA. The program would be phased in over perhaps a year.

Funding for the MSAs would come from savings generated by switching to low-cost/high-deductible policies. Catastrophic costs, such as surgeries for illness or accident, would be handled with traditional insurance provided by the employer via a traditional insurance carrier, but at an extremely inexpensive rate for say, $3,000–$5,000 deductible. (Currently a family of four may pay $400 to $600 per month, or approximately $5,000 to $7,000 per year. If average actual health-care costs are about $1,500 per year, three guesses at who keeps the profit!!!)

Americans want the best buy for their money. If the ER doc says there's very little chance of a serious underlying cause to your headache, then you'll be willing to take the two Percodan and call him in the morning, potentially averting the $1,400 charge that would have come from your own account. Of course, he may not offer you that option openly without tort reform.

ADVANTAGES OF MSAS

There are many potential advantages to a reform package centered on MSAs. The Private Medical Foundation of Shawnee, Oklahoma, points out the following eight:

1. Saving Money: People will purchase medical care with their MSA funds and thus be better shoppers.

2. Restore the doctor-patient relationship: The two individuals most concerned about an individual health problem work together to fix it without a bureaucrat or insurance company employee to guide them.

3. Maintain quality of care: MSAs would allow the marketplace to self-correct through free choice. The patient and physician together would choose the best course of action tailored individually to that case, not as "allowed" by a third party whose only concern is profit.

4. Encourage rationing by choice: Families and individuals would decide which monies would be spent on health care and which on other essentials.

5. Provide funds for preventive care: MSAs would be available for preventive exams and testing often not covered by insurance.

6. Provide for insurance premiums: MSAs accrued over time would provide for premiums during periods of unemployment.

7. Long-term care: MSA funds not expended during

working years would be available for Medicare supplement over age sixty-five.

8. Benefits personal and portable: MSAs would be private personal property and would go with the employee when jobs changed.[23]

If MSAs or their equivalent are not available through your employer and only managed-care options are offered, encourage your benefits personnel to avoid gatekeeper-insurance-owned systems at all costs. These systems are the most restrictive with respect to both patient choice and physician authority. Instead, seek out physician-owned, physician- run, multispecialty groups. While these groups may function on a "capitated" basis, they often avoid "gatekeeping" in the recognition that it fosters substandard care. Medical decisions with respect to quality assurance, outcome data, and diagnostic and therapeutic cost efficiencies are at least made by the ones who have the knowledge to make them, rather than paramedical financial personnel.

MEDICAID/MEDICARE

But our next problem, you will recall, is Medicaid/Medicare. This one won't be easy to fix. This behemoth must be contained by limiting the number of people who benefit from it. Many, many working people are on Medicaid, both legally and illegally. If the blue-collar worker could afford high-deductible insurance because of his MSA for routine costs, he wouldn't be on Medicaid. Perhaps affluent retirees who absolutely do not need Medicare could be suspended from benefits until such time as they could show that they do need it. (My parents will kill me for this one!)

True *urban* indigents currently have access to the best doctors and technology in the world via the state and county hospital system. Don't destroy this by decreasing funding at these levels. Shifting the care of the inner city indigent to all private facilities via anti-dumping laws just double taxes the working public by way of resultant cost-shifting and state and federal taxes. Expand the county hospital systems for care of the indigent. Support neighborhood clinics for delivery of preventive health care to this segment of the population. These are legitimate government expenditures.

Government MSAs and affordable catastrophic insurance will help the working poor, but the rural indigent are a different problem. True, much of the true indigent population gravitates to urban centers anyway because of the greater availability of assistance programs and job opportunities. The remaining rural poor may need to be part of a Medicaid program, but one that pays reasonably for services so as to avoid the hidden tax to us all of cost-shifting by institutions to their third-party payors. There may be a regulatory need with respect to guaranteeing rural indigents access to extensions of urban government-supported clinic systems. In any event, the reality of managed care medicine will drive some of the good physicians found in urban surplus to more rural locations where they may make less money but retain higher degrees of autonomy.

DEFENSIVE MEDICINE

Tort reform must be part of any legislative package. The entire premise of a market-force medical-industrial complex driven solely by the legitimate costs of delivering health care depends on eliminating the direct costs of malpractice premiums, but to a much greater extent, eliminating the need for defensive-medicine practices. Our young physicians are not even learning the difference between necessary testing and defensive testing. The emotional strain is driving many practicing physicians at the peak of their medical careers to seek alternate ways to make a living. This strain develops not only from constant attention to potential legal consequences, but from time and effort spent on massive piles of paperwork to file claims, acquiring precertification for everything (always from someone not as qualified as you to make the decision), and hours of meetings devoted to trying to fathom the current morass of partially managed managed care systems.

Why shouldn't plaintiff attorneys pay the legal costs of the defendant when they lose a case? If they're so sure that malpractice was committed, surely they should be willing to bear the costs of the case if they lose. No one's asking the plaintiff attorney to pay for the mental anguish and suffering of the unjustly accused physician and his family, but couldn't even the court costs be covered as in England and Japan?

Why can't the jury in a trial know of other compensation already received by the plaintiff when damages are being assessed? You know why: because the plaintiff attorney gets a huge percentage (usually 30–40 percent) of the award, that's why.

So why can't the attorney work for a fee just like I do, not on contingency? Can you see your doctor telling you that if he successfully removes your kidney he'll be taking a higher percentage of whatever we determine that kidney is worth to you?

Why is there not a cap on pain and suffering in all states instead of just a few? Does it seem right to put an arbitrary, astronomical value on an intangible, whether or not there exist covered medical expenses? In 1994, Democratic proposals before Congress actually suggested eliminating existing caps.

Is joint and several liability even constitutional? Just because I am associated with an individual or institution that is culpable for actions leading to an injury, should I be held just as accountable and punished? Am I my brother's keeper?

Should physicians be allowed a jury of their peers? If I study medicine for fifteen years, should an automotive plant worker be the one to decide, on the basis of purchased expert testimony, whether my actions were in error? When was it that we decided physicians aren't human and indeed are not allowed to make errors in judgment or otherwise?

TECHNOLOGY

Our fourth complicating factor that leads to high costs, you will recall, is the price of rapidly expanding high technology. Suppose an MRI machine costs two million dollars. What do you suppose the product liability in terms of research and development, superfluous manufacturing alterations to protect against unreal but perceived potential threats, and direct liability insurance premiums add to the cost of that MRI? Remember the headlines in 1993: someone has already successfully litigated for the loss of psychic ability during scanning.

The development of new pharmaceuticals and technologies with medical applications carries some unavoidable costs. But the leading drug companies should not be forced overseas in part because of legal costs near 30 percent of their net income. Tort reform must include laws that ease the burden of product liability on our manufacturing sector as well as on physicians and hospitals.

INFLATION

Inflation is clearly beyond the exclusive control of the government in a market society. While the Federal Reserve can act in what it perceives to be our best interest, there is probably little we can do to deal with this aspect of rising health-care costs. We can only recognize that this inflation annually magnifies the true rising cost of health care and, in effect, adds insult to injury. But in a similar fashion, the dollars saved by efficient reform are more valuable in an inflationary environment.

So, we have a problem. Not an insurmountable problem, for, I feel that, short of breaching the laws of Newtonian physics, nothing is impossible for the American people. If we recognize what is good about the system, eliminate what is bad, and make sure that we don't confuse the two, we can reduce the national costs and ensure at least adequate access for all.

But if we allow the government, the insurance industry, managed competition, or anyone else to destroy the physician-patient relationship, undermine the physician's authority to make decisions, and eliminate the patient's ability to choose, our health-care system will deteriorate to a level not seen in this century.

I don't honestly think the public realizes that the rewards we seek as physicians are really not only financial. Yes, while we think we should be well compensated for years and years of personal sacrifice and training well into early middle age, our true rewards come from the intimate involvement with the triumphs and tragedies of the lives of our patients. We became physicians because we realized that there are only a few ways in the short span of time available to us that we can touch the lives of those around us. And up to now it's been a ball!

Still, every doc I know is planning his alternative career, no kidding. My brother knows a forty-four-year-old general surgeon who just quit and opened a pizza parlor! I know of a plastic surgeon and his wife, an internist, who are planning to quit and teach high school. Another gynecologist at my hospital recently retired at forty-three and went into the computer software business. Another friend is considering quitting to raise cutting horses.

Lack of dedication, you say? I don't think so. Not after four years of college, four years of medical school, and three to seven years of residency. No, not lack of dedication, but lack of an attainable goal. Present circumstances are taking away the object of all those years of hard work. Managed competition will rob the physician of his most precious possession, his only true motivation. *It will rob him of his patient.*

Do not be confused by legislative debate on the national level. For the most part, it is the discussion of who will bear the brunt of the cost of expanding government's role in the delivery of health care. There are many eloquent published arguments debating universal coverage versus guaranteed coverage for single working moms and children, or debating the macroeconomic effect on our GNP of shifting an estimated $80 billion from upper income levels to lower, or debating the reasons behind the crumbling European socialized health-care systems, or any of a myriad of other predominantly economic debates about how the haves will pay for the health of the have-nots.[24] But for the most part, the insidious process of converting American medicine from a physician-driven to a provider-driven system is occurring without government intervention. We are allowing it to occur by giving away our authority to make our own choices when we allow a corporate third party to foot the bill.

Oh, medicine will continue no matter what. Lawyers

and insurance executives will continue to prosper from the new system. But if we're not careful, we won't have the best and the brightest at the other end of the stethoscope. We'll have a competent individual, happy to work from eight to five for the big company, caring not at all about patient rotation but valuing his job security and time off. In fact, we'll have just what the gentleman with the goatee at the managed-care seminar suggested, a medical system whose physicians deliver a commodity just like every other businessman.

So get ready. It's coming. Unless you take action to stop it *proactively,* you're going to give up yet another freedom. You're going to give up the freedom to choose who touches you in the most private ways, who cares for you when you're miserable, who listens to you when you're down, who rejoices with you when you're well. And even worse, you're going to create a system in which you may be lucky to find in a physician the virtues that once were requisite.

CONCLUSION

WHAT CAN YOU DO to preserve the finest health-care system in the world? What can you do to keep compassion alive in the doctor-patient relationship? First, here's what you don't have to do.

You don't have to understand the intricacies of the on-again, off-again debates that rage in Washington, because even many of those embroiled in them do not.

You don't have to understand the intricacies of the myriad different managed-competition paradigms that have been proposed as well as those already in existence.

You don't have to formulate your own plan for controlling health-care costs while expanding care for the needy.

Here's what you do have to do: Reject any scenario that restricts your choice of physician or facility.

If one of your insurance choices includes such restrictions, I can assure you that the participating physicians have substantially lost their decision-making authority. Your health care will then be controlled by a corporate entity whose sole motivation is to be profitable.

Insist that your employer research and offer plans that do not restrict choice, even if those plans require large deductibles or involve employers contracting directly with health-care systems. At the very least, the doctors from whom you currently receive care should be "grandfathered" for you in such a restrictive system. A choice with a large deductible may not seem financially possible on your income, but we know statistically that paying for your own routine health care out-of-pocket or out of money pooled and withheld by your employer *must* be cost-effective because the alternative, which includes filing a claim on relatively small outlays, generates huge profits for the insurers.

Women, don't allow yourself to be forced into a situation in which you do not have direct access to your OB/GYN. You may have looked years before finding the doctor with whom you are really comfortable. As mentioned previously, 90 percent of your health problems under

185

age fifty will fall within the expertise of your OB/GYN. There is no reason to accept an insurance plan of any sort that forces you to see a physician other than your OB/GYN for your routine care or gynecologic problems.

Managed care in some form is probably here to stay. If it is truly your only financially possible option, then look for systems with no "gatekeeper" component. Large multispecialty, physician-run HMOs *not* built on a gatekeeper model are more likely to deliver quality care, even if fully capitated, by avoiding the scenario whereby a screening physician decides if and/or which specialist you are permitted to see.

I urge women to write to their state legislators and support legislation that would mandate insurers granting unrestricted access to their OB/GYNs at *least* once per year. California, Delaware, Georgia, Maryland, New York, and Virginia are the only states as of this writing that have passed some such legislation.

Some state legislatures are learning the hard way. In May 1995 the Washington State legislature repealed almost every provision of its once vaunted "universal coverage" health care, which was virtually identical to the Clinton proposal. They threw out, by veto-proof majorities, employer mandates, mandated managed-care guidelines, and a state commission's power to micro-manage healthcare.

Our legislators should concentrate their efforts on plans that address only the indigent and working uninsured. Leave the rest of the system alone. They should give whatever incentives possible to small businesses who self-insure. Pooled withholdings to pay for outlays that fall into the deductible range of inexpensive catastrophic policies should be tax-free to the individual.

Our nationwide county hospital/clinic system should be actively underwritten by the federal government. It is a mistake to cripple these academic institutions by placing them in direct unrestricted competition with private hospitals involved in managed-care contracting. Competition not only endangers excellent care now available to indigents, it directly threatens the survival of our country's university hospitals and graduate medical-education programs. Neighborhood clinics involved in preventive health care should be expanded in all our metropolitan areas, and ties to their associated university system strengthened.

Reform and or federal regulation of the insurance industry is far beyond the scope of this text. However, *legislators should meet tomorrow and mandate the removal of all preexisting-condition exclusions.* It is cruel. It is wrong. The burden could be equitably distributed to all of the companies in the industry. Furthermore, policies should be portable. A job change should not affect an individual's health coverage unless the new job involves handling Uranium 238, waving red towels in front of angry bulls, or running tests on the Ebola virus. We could restore a little compassion right there.

The world community still views health care in the United States as the best available anywhere. I firmly believe the success of our system is rooted in the doctor-patient relationship. It is the joy of the art of healing that drives great minds, great medical education, and great research. If we destroy the joy of medicine for the physician, take away his relationship to the patient, and afford him the same position in the national psyche as any other worker, we will lose more than we ever thought possible.

In this great country, freedom of choice, whether related to speech, religion, education, or health care, is the foundation of our success. *Any proposals that significantly restrict your freedom to choose must be vigorously opposed.* The ideas put forth that limit your choice are the same ones that undermine the decision-making authority of our society's trained health professionals.

We must let neither the government nor our insurance companies undermine our liberty. In 1928, Justice Louis Brandeis said, "Experience should teach us to be most on our guard to protect our liberty when the government's [or insurance companies'] purposes are beneficent. The greatest dangers to liberty lurk in the insidious encroachment by men of zeal, well meaning, but without understanding."[25]

1. *ACOG Technical Bulletins* 1995
2. Kassberg, Maria, "Turf War" in *OBG Management,* October 1994, pg. 46
3. Ibid, pg. 53
4. "NCI Changes Its Stance," *JAMA,* 271(2):96, Jan. 12, 1994
5. Miller, A.B., et al, Canadian National Breast Cancer Screening Study, *Canadian Med. Assoc. Jrnl.* 147:1459–1476, 1992
6. Kerlilowsky, K., et al, "Positive Predictive Value of Screening Mammography by Age," *JAMA* 270:2444–2450, 1993
7. Smigel, U., et al, "Canadian Mammogram Study to be Reviewed," *Jrnl. of NCI,* 87 (6): 413, March 1995
8. Shapiro, S., "Efficacy of Screening Mammogram," *Jrnl. of NCI,* 86(22): 1722, and discussion 1722–25, November 1994
9. Greenberg, D.S., "NCI Blasted for Mammography Confusion," *Lancet* 344(8933):1353, November 1994
10. Osuch, J, et al, "Mammography Guidelines," Ca: *Cancer Jrnl. for Clinicians,* 44(5):319, 1994
11. Parker, M.D., Steve, "Digital Stereotactic and Whole Breast Mammography," presented at Breast Cancer Update 1995, PHD, Feb. 3, 1995
12. Sickles, E.A., "Mammographic Screening," *Annals of Internal Medicine,* 122(7):534–8, Apr. 1, 1995
13. Vogel, V.G., Monographs—NCI (16):55–60, 1994
14. Kassirer, J., "Academic Medicine Under Siege," *NEJM* Vol. 331:1370–1371, 1994
15. Page, Leigh, *AMA News,* Oct. 10, 1994
16. Jones, Del, "Election Gives Hospital Giant More Clout," *USA Today,* November 11, 1994, pg. B-1
17. Ibid, pg. B-2
18. Slomski, Anita, "How Business Is Flattening Health Costs," *Medical Economics,* August 1994, pg. 2
19. Ibid, pg. 5
20. Ibid, pg. 6
21. Swartz, Mimi, "Not What the Doctor Ordered," *Texas Monthly,* March 1995, pg. 116
22. Ibid, pg. 115
23. "Eight Advantages of MSAs," *Physicians for Patient Power Newsletter,* September 1994
24. Reinhardt, "Coverage and Access in Health Care Reform," *NEJM,* Vol. 330, No. 20, May 19, 1994, pg. 1452
25. Quoted by Head, Mark, in "The Two Minute Drill for Health Reform," August 11, 1994

*(from page 142) Most HMOs do not permit themselves to be sued for malpractice. All patients, as part of their contracts, must sign and agree to binding arbitration, even if unknowingly.